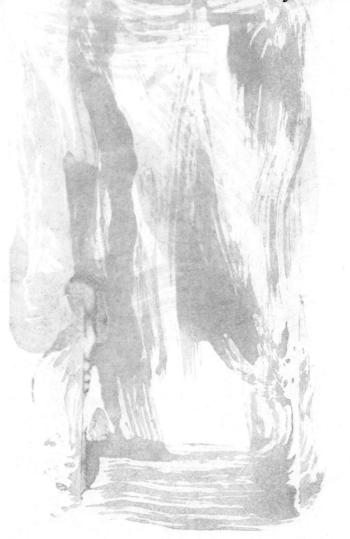

Physiology and pathophysiology
of the body fluids

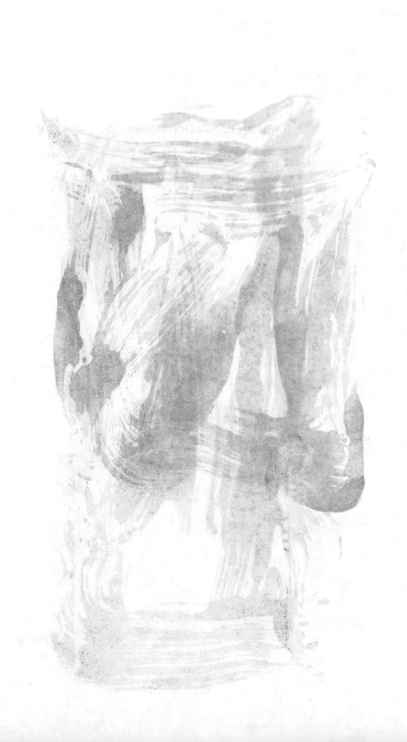

Physiology and pathophysiology of the body fluids

MAUREEN WIMBERLY GROËR, M.S.N., Ph.D.

Associate Professor, University of Tennessee
College of Nursing, Knoxville, Tennessee

with 65 *illustrations*

The C. V. Mosby Company

ST. LOUIS • TORONTO • LONDON   1981

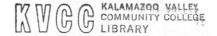

MOSBY

1906 **75** 1981
YEARS

A TRADITION OF PUBLISHING EXCELLENCE

Editor: Thomas Allen Manning
Manuscript editor: Sue Jane Smith
Designer: Jeanne Bush
Production: Jeanne Gulledge

Printed in the United States of America

The C. V. Mosby Company
11830 Westline Industrial Drive, St. Louis, Missouri 63141

Library of Congress Cataloging in Publication Data

Groër, Maureen E   1944-
    Physiology and pathophysiology of the body
fluids.

    Bibliography: p.
    Includes index.
    1. Body fluids.   2. Body fluid disorders—
Nursing.   I. Title. [DNLM: 1. Water-electrolyte
imbalance.   2. Water-electrolyte balance.
3. Acid-base imbalance.   WD 220 G874p]
QP90.5.G76   616.3'9   80-28583
ISBN 0-8016-1989-0

GW/D/D 9 8 7 6 5 4 3 2 1   02/C/257

Contributors

MARY ELLEN BANKS, R.N., M.S.N. *Chapter 12*

Assistant Professor, University of Tennessee College of Nursing,
Knoxville, Tennessee

DALE GOODFELLOW, R.N., Ph.D. *Chapter 4 case study*

Associate Professor, University of Tennessee College of Nursing,
Knoxville, Tennessee

LINDA LAW HARRISON, R.N., M.S.N. *Chapter 11 case study*

Instructor, University of Tennessee College of Nursing,
Knoxville, Tennessee

JUNE MARTIN, R.N. *Chapter 9 case study*

RANDALL MAUPIN, R.N., M.S.N. *Chapter 8 case study*

Instructor, University of Tennessee College of Nursing,
Knoxville, Tennessee

CAROLYN McDONOUGH SAMPSELLE, R.N., M.S.N.
Chapter 11 case study

Assistant Professor, University of Tennessee College of Nursing,
Knoxville, Tennessee

Preface

This book has been written for students and practitioners of nursing who believe that an understanding of normal physiology is an absolute necessity before fluids, electrolytes, acids, and bases can be understood. A physiologic approach is used in this book so that the reader will gain an understanding of normal function and thus be able to predict the signs and symptoms of imbalance.

I have used several case studies as illustrative examples of imbalance throughout the book. These studies were derived from the histories of patients for whom my colleagues and I have cared in clinical settings.

An additional approach in this book is an integration of physical assessment skills that are necessary so that the nurse can adequately care for patients with fluid, electrolyte, or acid-base imbalances. It has been assumed in the text that the reader is familiar with the actual techniques of physical assessment. The text provides information on how to use these techniques in the care of patients and describes the common findings of the physical assessment in clients with various imbalances.

I would like to acknowledge my colleagues who contributed case studies and valuable suggestions during the writing of this book. Their names and contributions are listed separately. My family, as always, has been self-sacrificing and understanding, and my love for them cannot be expressed.

Maureen Wimberly Groër

Contents

1

Physical laws and physiologic processes influencing fluids, electrolytes, acids, and bases

Man is a particularly well adapted creature. What other animal, through modern technology, can travel in a few hours' time from one climate to another climate that is completely different and still maintain his body temperature, his internal water environment, and the concentrations of the various dissolved substances in his body fluids? Man can regulate his internal body environment through biologic mechanisms that have developed through evolutionary processes as well as through intelligent manipulation of both the environment and his own physiology.

Man maintains homeostasis, or the *steady state*, through these biologic mechanisms, which respond when the external environment changes. Without this regulation, man's fluid and electrolyte balance would quickly change, resulting in an equilibrium of the internal environment with the external environment. No concentration differences in the various body compartments could be maintained. The chemicals that make up the body fluids would return to the external environment from which they originally came, and man as a unique structural and functional entity would cease to exist.

Evolutionary theory implies that a species retains characteristics that confer selective survival advantages. These characteristics arise through mutations in the species gene pool. Those members of the species with traits that allow them to live longer, healthier lives, and to breed more often than other members, are destined to pass their genetic traits on to more offspring. The regulatory mechanisms that maintain the constancy of the internal body environment have evolved through natural selection, and they allow man to function optimally in a manner well adapted to his environment. The original living organisms were unicellular and probably had an internal environment that was extremely similar to that of the fluid in which they lived. Through the process of natural selection the more complex living creatures gradually evolved a highly specialized internal milieu that became greatly different from the world around them. This environment, which of course allows the organism a greater complexity of activities and behaviors, nevertheless requires an extraordinary amount of genetic control, regulation, and energy utilization.

Of additional import to an understanding of fluid and electrolyte integrity in man is the fact that since the industrial revolution man has changed his external environment so significantly that these same mechanisms that allow for coping and adaptation may no longer be functional. Man also faces a future in which the possibility of manipulation of his internal environment, through drugs and genetic control, may be the only way that man can survive in a new and hostile physicochemical world.

REGULATORY PROCESSES

The many mechanisms that regulate the body's internal environment do not function alone but in an integrated manner with other types of physiologic regulation, thus the organism as a whole acts in a unified manner when presented with environmental change. Furthermore the human organism is able to effect internal constancy through many different processes, a phenomenon known as *equifinality*. A salt and fluid load on the normal physiology will trigger many adaptive and regulatory mechanisms. Adaptive measures allow the organism to cope with change in the normal volume and electrolyte concentration, whereas regulatory mechanisms act to eliminate excess fluid and salt so that total body water and salt return to normal, or steady state, values. Examples of adaptive measures include several cardiovascular reflexes that act to preserve the function of the system. Examples of the regulatory mechanisms include neurologic reflexes that act to decrease thirst and increase urine output. There are, of course, many systemic reflexes that are both adaptive and regulatory.

Physiologic regulation is achieved mainly through *feedback* mechanisms. Feedback—the major way that internal constancy is continuously achieved—is essential because the concentration of the various dissolved substances in the body fluids must be carefully controlled within an ex-

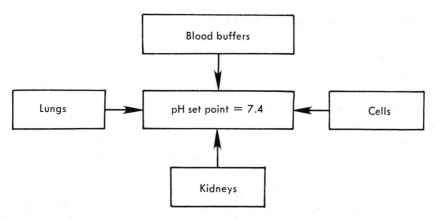

Fig. 1-1. Normal pH set point of 7.4 is maintained through interaction of four major buffering systems: when pH changes, various "sensors" immediately respond to initiate buffering and return pH to normal.

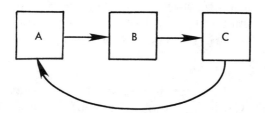

Fig. 1-2. In end-product inhibition, end product, C, increases in production up to a certain value (set point) and inhibits reaction $A \rightarrow B$.

tremely limited range around the normal mean values. Thus the regulatory feedback systems somehow are able to "know" what is normal and to "sense" what is abnormal. The normal value for a feedback regulatory system is known as the *set point*. For example, the pH of the blood is usually 7.4. When this value changes, various physiologic processes are instantly activated to adjust the pH back to the normal value. Thus the set point is that value above or below which regulatory feedback systems are activated. Fig. 1-1 presents this concept in more detail.

The importance of constant feedback by which information is supplied to a regulatory or adaptive system cannot be emphasized enough to the student of fluid and electrolyte physiology. The information can be supplied as either negative or positive feedback. An example of negative feedback is end-product inhibition, as illustrated in Fig. 1-2. The end product of a physiologic process acts to turn off the initial steps in the process when the set point for the system is achieved. In the example previously given, when an excess fluid or salt load is present, a great number of feedback mechanisms sense the changes and activate a variety of processes that adjust the water and salt concentrations. When the normal values are returned, the set point is once again reached and the regulatory mechanisms are inactivated. Such systems often show an *overshoot* phenomenon, in which regulation results in the production of a value that is slightly greater than the true set point. This phenomenon is believed to act as a kind of "safety valve." It also results in another important phenomenon—the fluctuations that occur around mean values. Thus a range around a mean value is often considered normal. For example, the range of blood pH is usually stated to be between 7.35 and 7.45.

Positive feedback, the second type of physiologic control, acts by means of end-product stimulation of earlier steps. Thus it acts in a self-enhancing or self-perpetuating manner to continually propagate a process, a chemical substance, or another parameter. Negative feedback plays the major role in fluid and electrolyte physiology, whereas positive feedback often develops during pathophysiologic processes.

COMPARTMENTS

Another important concept in fluid and electrolyte physiology is that of compartments. Man is a multicompartmented system. This statement implies that the fluids contained within the body do not mix freely but are constrained by the various membrane-enclosed spaces that exist. The cell, for example, is a fluid compartment, and collectively all the fluid within cells forms a compartment known as the intracellular fluid (ICF). Extracellular fluid (ECF) is also a compartment and is further divided into many smaller subcompartments. Compartments of ECF include plasma, joint fluids, cerebrospinal fluid, and so forth.

The many fluid compartments are separated anatomically and physiologically, but nevertheless an exchange is possible between these compartments. Constant control of the contents of each compartment is therefore a necessary part of fluid physiology. Fluid compartments are generally separated from other parts of the body by membranes.

It is also possible to speak of compartments of *solutes*. For example, within a structure there may be several sodium compartments. One compartment may be exchangeable with the environment, but a second may be sequestered and unavailable. These solute compartments are prob-

ably more physiologic than anatomic, although there is always an inter-
play of both in any function.

To clearly describe the fluid and electrolyte compartments, it is necessary to review basic physiologic concepts that determine the nature and
function of the various compartments.

CELL MORPHOLOGY AND PHYSIOLOGY

All the cells of the body are modified from four basic types: epithelial,
connective, nervous, and muscle. These cells become differentiated during
normal embryonic development and are different both structurally and
functionally. Figs. 1-3 to 1-6 illustrate these different cell types as they
appear under the microscope.

The structure and function of the basic cell types have great relevance
to fluid and electrolyte balance and imbalance. For example, a knowledge
of the cell types of the epidermis and dermis will provide a background
for skin assessment in dehydration. An understanding of nerve structure is necessary for a full appreciation of how electrolyte imbalances
alter excitability and transmission.

Epithelial cells are found as part of the lining of most membranes.
They are often secretory in nature and are often continuously shed from

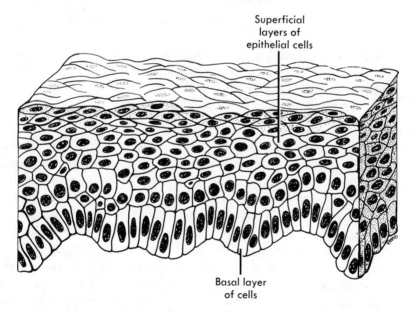

Superficial
layers of
epithelial cells

Basal layer
of cells

Fig. 1-3. Stratified squamous epithelium such as lines mouth.

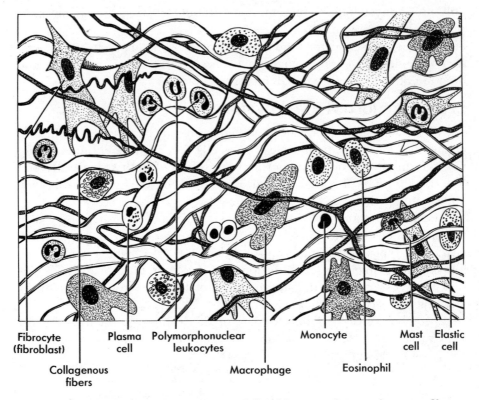

Fibrocyte
(fibroblast)
Plasma
cell
Polymorphonuclear
leukocytes
Monocyte
Mast
cell
Elastic
cell
Collagenous
fibers
Macrophage
Eosinophil

Fig. 1-4. Areolar connective tissue. Several fibroblasts can be seen between fibers. Note also macrophages, plasma cell, mast cell, and three types of white blood cells: polymorphonuclear leukocytes, eosinophils, and monocyte.

the surface and replaced by new like cells. These cells may be found as a single layer as in the capillary endothelium, or they may be arranged in layers as in the skin. The appearance of the skin epithelium under the microscope is stratified, and the basal layer of cells, which consists of dividing replacement cells, is gradually replaced by square, flat squamous cells as the cells approach the surface of the epithelium and then die there and are sloughed off. The water content of epithelial cells decreases as the cells move from the basal layer to the surface.

Connective tissue acts to cushion and protect organs and to give vessels and other structures a certain degree of rigidity and form. Connective tissue makes up cartilage and bone as well, and the blood is also considered a type of connective tissue. The prominent features of all connective tissue are (1) cells, (2) fibers, and (3) matrix, or ground substance,

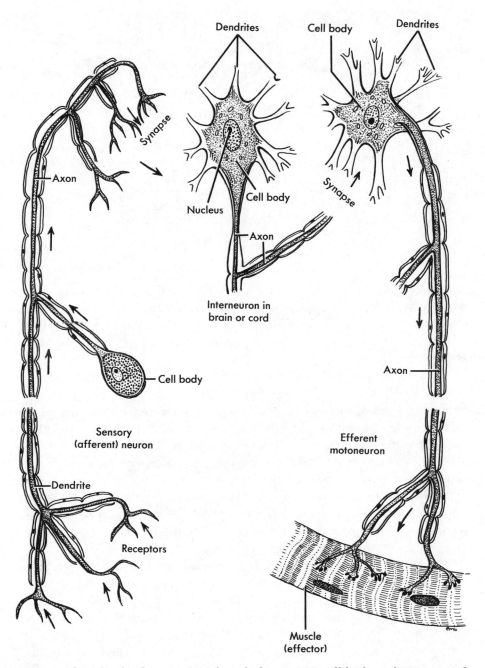

Fig. 1-5. Three kinds of neurons, each with three parts: cell body and two types of extensions, dendrite(s) and axon. Note direction of impulse conduction *(arrows).*

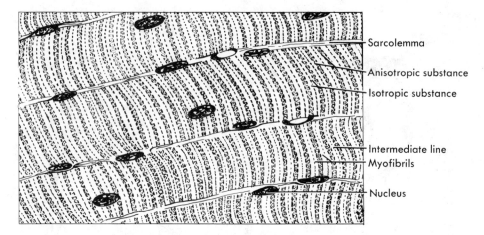

Fig. 1-6. Skeletal (striated, voluntary) muscle tissue.

in which the cells and fibers lie. The different types of cells elaborate proteins such as collagen, fibrin, and elastin, which then form the actual fibers that are largely responsible for the consistency of the tissue. Connective tissue contains a high proportion of water and often actually secretes fluid.

Nervous tissue consists of nerve cells that are extremely well differentiated, rarely, if ever, dividing after the first year of life in the human. Nerve cells make multiple connections, or synapses, with other nerve cells, muscles, glands, and other structures. Within the brain and spinal cord these masses of nerve cells are supported by connective tissue and glial cells. Some nerve cells are myelinated, being coated with many rings of a lipidlike substance that acts to protect and insulate the inner cytoplasm of the cell and to allow electrochemical changes to travel unimpeded down the length of the nerve cell processes. Nervous tissue containing many myelinated fibers appears white in contrast to the gray appearance of unmyelinated nervous tissue.

Muscle tissue is the fourth unique tissue type and consists of three major types: skeletal, smooth, and cardiac. Skeletal muscle is innervated by motor nerves and can be consciously controlled. Its function is to allow movement of the bones and joints. Smooth muscle is involuntary, although biofeedback research has demonstrated that some degree of conscious control can be achieved over the activity of some smooth and cardiac muscle. Smooth muscle lines hollow viscera such as the bladder, the gastrointestinal tract, and the ureters. Smooth muscle also lines all the blood vessels except the capillaries. The innervation of smooth muscle is through the autonomic nervous system, which consists of the sympathetic and parasympathetic divisions. Nervous supply is not absolutely necessary for contraction, however, since both smooth and cardiac muscle possess the property of *automaticity*. Such muscle can contract entirely without nervous or endocrine influence, and it usually contracts in a rhythmic, genetically determined pattern and rate.

Cardiac muscle is found only in the heart and is structurally and functionally more like smooth muscle than skeletal muscle. Cardiac muscle is *syncytial* in nature, although not in structure. A syncytium consists of a group of cells that act in a unified manner, responding to change in any member of the syncytium in the same way. Cardiac muscle thus responds to a depolarizing event in a cardiac cell, which then initiates a wave of depolarization throughout the heart. Some syncytia (skeletal muscle) are so well developed that the individual cells have lost their membrane, and a giant, multinucleated cell is thus formed.

All muscle tissue is well differentiated and, like nerve tissue, rarely divides. Injury to both nerve and muscle results in healing through the replacement of the damaged tissue by connective tissue, which ultimately forms a scar. Healing of epithelial tissue may result in repair of the defect with identical cells, and thus no scar is formed. The parenchyma of organs such as the liver and kidney is epithelial in nature, and such organs have remarkable properties of regeneration when injured. This is not true of muscle or nerve tissue.

Thus it can be seen that all tissues and their cells are vastly different from one another, and that even within a given organ, many different tissue types act together to maintain functional integrity. For example, an organ such as the kidney has a connective tissue capsule and stroma; an epithelial matrix; a vascular supply of epithelium, connective tissue, and smooth muscle; and a nervous supply as well. The major cell types of the body are nevertheless very similar in some respects. For example, all cells contain nuclei and organelles and are bounded by a cell membrane, all cells contain water as the principal constituent, and all cells perform cellular work to adjust the electrolyte concentrations of the various solutes contained within them. Therefore the next section of this chapter will describe the commonalities of cell biology, particularly with regard to fluids and electrolytes. The regulation of the latter is ultimately carried out by cells, and the basis of the regulation resides in (1) the particular dependencies of the various cell types on certain electrolytes and other molecules and (2) the ability of the cells to sense alterations and respond through metabolic work to the challenge of regulation.

The three basic components of a mammalian cell—membrane, cytoplasm, and nucleus—are greatly modified in the different cell types, depending on the function of the cell. The cell membrane of a secretory cell, for example, can be seen to be extraordinarily active when viewed with the electron microscope. The cell membrane components are continuously being renewed, and the cell surface is highly folded. Many vesicles containing a cell's particular secretion are budded off from the surface in membrane enclosures. Nuclear activity is also dependent on the cell type and on the current stage in the cell cycle. Since nerve cells, for example, do not engage in mitosis, the activity of the deoxyribonucleic acid (DNA) is limited to protein synthesis. Other cell types undergo constant mitotic turnover, when members of the cell compartment are lost and must be replaced, as in the skin. Thus these replacement cells, or stem cells, are mitotically active, and under the microscope one can see many mitotic spindles in which the cell's chromosomes are lined up and pulled apart into two new daughter cells. Depending on function, some cells appear to be very active metabolically. Thus liver cells contain many more mitochondria than skin cells, since the liver is a major organ of metabolic processes and control. Large amounts of work are done by these cells, which therefore require increased amounts of adenosine triphosphate (ATP), which is supplied through the mitochondrial metabolism of glucose. Thus it can be seen that the structure and function of different cells become greatly modified by both the cell's type and its environment.

Cell membrane

Perhaps no other structure assumes as much importance in fluid and electrolyte physiology as the cell membrane. To maintain the fluid and electrolyte compartments of the body, the cell membrane must be able to regulate the movement of fluids and solutes. The structure of the mammalian cell membrane is presently the subject of considerable research. Early models of the membrane described it as a "fat sandwich," with two layers of fat (or lipid) sandwiched between layers of protein. This model is depicted in Fig. 1-7 as it was originally devised by Danielli and Davson. Recent work having clarified the structure of the membrane, it is now known that the membrane forms a lipoprotein mosaic, as illustrated in Fig. 1-8. Thus the membrane contains a bilayer of lipid oriented

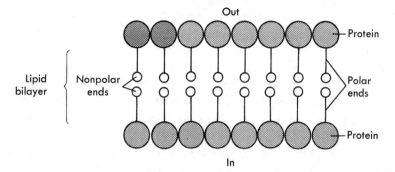

Fig. 1-7. Model of membrane depicting, cell membrane's being coated on outer and inner surfaces with a layer of protein. Interior is composed of hydrophobic core of lipid, oriented as bilayer, with nonpolar ends facing interior of membrane.

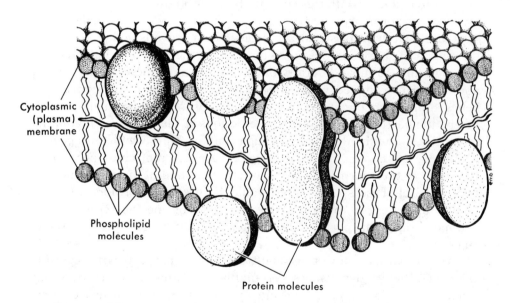

Fig. 1-8. Possible structure of cytoplasmic and internal cell membranes. Membrane's molecular structure consists of (1) bilayer of phospolipid molecules arranged with their "tails" pointing toward each other and (2) protein molecules located in all possible positions in relation to phospholipid bilayer—at outer surface, at inner surface, partially penetrating bilayer, and extending completely through membrane.

so that the hydrophilic (water-loving) ends of the molecules are oriented toward the outside, and the hydrophobic (water-hating) ends face toward the inside, making up an internal hydrophobic core. Protein does coat the lipid on both sides of the hydrophobic core, but protein is also interspersed with lipid and can actually go through the entire width of the membrane. The lipid and protein appear to be arranged to allow for previously unexplained membrane functions. For example, protein enables the membrane to assume certain molecular configurations that make up receptor sites for the many hundreds of molecules that both interact with cells and affect them. Antigen-binding sites, hormone receptors, virus receptors, complement-binding sites, and so forth all require a certain specific membrane stereochemistry. Such stereochemistry was difficult to explain with the model of the membrane as devised by Danielli and Davson. Cell membranes also transport solutes across the membrane in both inward and outward directions. Molecules that are somehow free to move within the lipid matrix of the membrane are a requirement of such transport. The former idea of a rigid bilayer was difficult to reconcile with this concept. It is now known that the cell membrane is extraordinarily active. Some of the molecules that make up its structure have half-lives that are measured in seconds. Other studies of the membrane have demonstrated that within the lipid matrix many proteins are able to move laterally or to flip-flop, and these properties are now being investigated with regard to various forms of transport. It is believed also that the structure of the membrane is continuously modified by the particular physiologic interactions of the cells with regulating molecules and with other cells, through contact. Thus a cell's surface may at one period consist of many specific receptor molecules because of induction of their formation by an interaction, and at another time perhaps none of these specific sites would be present. Hormones, in particular, appear able to induce the formation of specific receptor sites and membrane transport capabilities for a variety of transportable molecules.

Cell membranes may occasionally function improperly with regard to transport. Dietary deficiencies, certain disease states, or some drugs may modify the surface greatly and alter normal transport. An extreme example is the massive increase in water permeability of erythrocytes occurring after envenomization with certain snake venoms. The venoms contain enzymes that destroy the normal bonds of the membrane phospholipids, causing large pores to appear in the membrane. Water leaks into the cell in great amounts and hemoglobin leaks out, a process called *hemolysis*. When hemolysis occurs, the erythrocytes are eventually destroyed, the hemoglobin is no longer able to transport oxygen, and cellular oxygenation and metabolism cannot occur. Although this example is dramatic, there are many drugs, diseases, and nutritional deficiencies that alter erythrocyte permeability to a lesser degree. Such cells are very fragile. Transit through the circulation can result in sequestering of these cells in the fairly hypoxic spleen, which leads to their hemolysis. Mechanical injury of these cells in capillaries throughout the body may occur as well, with resultant hemolysis. It should be apparent that for cells to function normally, the functional and structural integrity of the cell membrane lipoprotein mosaic is a necessity.

An important concept in membrane physiology is the idea that pores exist. It was formerly believed that molecules crossing the membrane traveled exclusively through pores of appropriate size and charge. The diffusion of substances from a higher concentration to a lower concentration thus would require a selectively permeable membrane—one that was able to selectively allow only certain substances to cross. Pore dimensions have been calculated for the movement of ions such as sodium and potassium. It is likely that some actual pores do exist within membranes, but for many ions and molecules that move across membranes, it would appear that carrier molecules are often involved, even for substances that cross the membrane by diffusion. A carrier molecule would allow the membrane to be very selective in transport because the size and charge of a pore would not be the only determinants. The actual mechanics of molecular movement across cell membranes will be discussed later, but it is necessary here to point out this special characteristic of membranes, which is the subject of much current research.

An additional feature of the cell membrane lies in its ability to separate charge and thus act like a battery. Charge separation is carried out by both the physicochemical permeability of the membrane and the active transport processes that maintain chemical gradients across the membrane. Most mammalian cells have some potential differences developed across their membranes, with nerve and muscle cells having the greatest voltage differences. The cell membrane is negatively charged with respect to the outside, and it is of course this property that allows nerve and muscle tissue to become excited and conductive. The development of the cell membrane potential and the characteristics of cell excitation will be discussed later in this book. Fluid and electrolyte physiology and pathophysiology become understandable only when a comprehension of the dynamics of the cell membrane potential is achieved.

Nucleus

The nucleus of each cell contains the genetic code in the form of molecules of DNA. The ultimate permeability of the cell membrane is determined by the DNA because the structure and function of the membrane are derived from the types and amounts of various enzymes and proteins formed by the cell. The cellular receptor sites, the transporting molecules, the enzymatic machinery for active transport of substances, and the components of membrane that must constantly be replaced as membrane material is lost or renewed are all coded for by the specific base sequences of a particular cell's active DNA. Fig. 1-9 shows the typical mammalian cell cycle of DNA activity.

The function of DNA is of course to translate into specific proteins through the process of protein synthesis and to permit the cell to undergo cell division, or mitosis, and thus to perpetuate the cell line. Fig. 1-9 shows that this period of mitosis is rather short compared to the synthetic phase of the cell cycle and to the long resting phases. In mitosis the chromosomes of the cell condense into distinct structures and line up in the middle of the cell. They are subsequently split into homologous halves, which move to opposite poles of the cell, and eventually into the daughter cells that are formed. The end result of mitosis is the formation of two genetically identical new cells. Active protein synthesis is carried out during the S phase of the cell cycle. Cells at this stage of the cycle consist of nuclei containing highly dispersed DNA, and no distinct chromosomal structures are visible. During protein synthesis certain segments of the DNA code, through enzymatic mechanisms, form complementary strands of ribonucleic acid (RNA). The RNA molecules, in turn, move into the cytoplasm of the cell, and some line up along the ribosomes, which are the actual site of protein synthesis. Other RNA molecules act to bind specific amino acids to them and are then transported to the ribosomes.

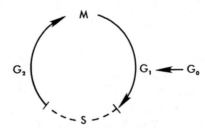

Fig. 1-9. Cell cycle: M represents phase during which mitosis occurs, G_1 and G_2 are phases between M and S (protein-synthesis phase), and G_0 is the resting phase.

The sequence of bases along the length of the RNA molecule determines which amino acids should be linearly arranged to ultimately form a protein strand.

The nature of the proteins that are coded for by DNA determines ultimately both the morphologic features and the functions of a cell. For example, liver cells will normally produce only liver proteins. The genes coding for all the other proteins produced in the human body are present in the liver cell (and all other cells), but these genes are repressed. If liver cells began to produce insulin or hemoglobin, the entire nature of the cell would be altered. When the cell is required to synthesize large amounts of a particular protein, the DNA code can be derepressed by certain proteins and through hormonal activity. An example of this phenomenon, called induction, which plays a role in fluid and electrolyte physiology, is the induction of a sodium *permease* by the hormone aldosterone. The synthesis of the permease protein appears to allow increased reabsorption of sodium ions at the distal convoluted tubule (DCT) in the nephrons of the kidney.

Cytoplasm

The cell cytoplasm is the matrix within which the biochemistry of the cell is allowed to proceed. It is thought of as a gel-like fluid, the viscosity and chemical nature of which can change as the cell so requires. Cellular motility, for example, may be permitted through a phenomenon known as sol-gel transformation, whereby projections of the cell extend outward and the internal cytoplasm gels. The cell moves forward as the cytoplasm inside the projections liquefies and then gels once again. For such activity to occur, the cellular water must stay constant. States of increased or decreased total body water ultimately may alter such processes as cell motility.

The cytoplasm contains organelles, which are discrete structures such as mitochondria, lysosomes, ribosomes, Golgi complex, and centrioles. The extent of development and number of the various organelles depend on the function of the cell. Liver cells, which are highly metabolic, contain many mitochondria. Secretory cells, on the other hand, contain a well-developed ribosomal system (the rough endoplasmic reticulum). Phagocytic cells such as leukocytes have many lysosomes, which are membrane-enclosed organelles containing hydrolytic enzymes. Phagocytic cells first engulf particulate matter, immune complexes, and bacteria and then enzymatically destroy or detoxify ingested material through reactions of the lysosomal enzymes.

Although cells differ greatly in structure and function, what has been described is the basic characteristics of all cells: membrane, nucleus, and cytoplasm. (The human erythrocyte is therefore not a true cell but a corpuscle, since it lacks a nucleus.)

When various deviations from the normal fluid, electrolyte, and pH values are discussed in this text, the alterations in normal cellular function and structure will be described. Many deviations, although ultimately having profound effects on normal organ and system physiology, nevertheless cause initial disruptions at the cellular level.

BASIC PHYSICAL AND PHYSIOLOGIC TRANSPORT MECHANISMS

Before the nature of the body water and the various compartments that compose it are described, the transport mechanisms of cell membranes will be discussed to aid in developing an understanding of compartmentalization. All compartments are membrane bound and thus are kept distinct through the unique properties of the membranes.

Diffusion

The diffusion of atoms, ions, or molecules occurs independently of any biologic process. Diffusion is the natural tendency of a substance to move from an area of higher concentration to one of lower concentration. Substances that are diffusing therefore move down their concentration gradients, or more simply, in a *downhill* direction. Diffusion is due to the natural, disordered, random movement of atoms and molecules in a solution. Since random movement of a concentrated solute will result in a greater *probability* of the solute's moving into the area of lesser concentration, an eventual equilibrium will be reached. It should be clear that random (or entropic) movement of solute molecules that enter the dilute solution will also occur. Since there are fewer molecules in the dilute solution, however, the overall tendency of the system is for the solute to move downhill until equilibrium is reached. Equilibrium is not a static state, however. At equilibrium there will be no overall concentration gradient for the solute; the random movements of the solute molecules will continue but will be equal in all directions (Fig. 1-10).

When two solutions of different solute concentrations are separated by a membrane, the tendency for diffusion will of course still be present. Nevertheless, in biologic systems, diffusion requires two variables: (1) a concentration gradient of a solute and (2) a selectively permeable mem-

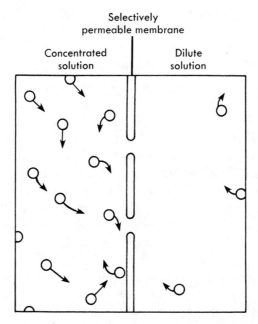

Fig. 1-10. Diffusion through selectively permeable membrane is result of greater probability that cell membrane will have contact with molecules of more concentrated solution.

brane that will permit the solute to move. Thus cell membranes can control what substances move into or out of the cell.

It is apparent in Fig. 1-10 that the cell membrane separating the two solutions will have a much greater *probability* of contact with the molecules making up solution A, which is highly concentrated. If as the molecules strike the membrane when they move entropically, there are pores or carrier molecules in the membrane, there will be a *net* tendency of the molecules to move through the membrane in a downhill direction. Some molecules from solution B will move uphill because an occasional molecule will happen to make contact with the membrane. Thus diffusion is the *net* movement of molecules down a concentration gradient. As increasing numbers of molecules from solution A move into solution B, there will be a loss of solute from A and a gain of solute in B. Eventually a point is reached where the concentration of solution A equals that of solution B. This is the equilibrium point. Equal movement in both directions then occurs across the membrane.

Net diffusion will be increased when the membrane is highly permeable to the solute that is diffusing or when the concentration gradient is very steep.

Regulation of membrane permeability is a physiologic process, whereas the steepness of the concentration gradient is a purely physical phenomenon. Membrane permeability to various diffusible substances is (1) a function of the different lipids that make up the membrane as well as various membrane proteins and (2) a result of the nature of pores and carriers. Many substances that diffuse easily through the cell membrane are soluble in lipid. Gases such as carbon dioxide and oxygen are good examples. These gases diffuse very rapidly, whereas other substances, such as Na^+, K^+, and other ions, are much more soluble in water than in an oily solution. The fact that ethanol rapidly diffuses through lipid accounts for its extremely fast uptake from the stomach into the blood. Substances that are lipid soluble dissolve more or less through the membrane lipid down the concentration gradient. Substances that are not lipid soluble generally are more restricted in their diffusion and must move through channels or be transported by carrier molecules.

Diffusion through pores or channels is the common mechanism for most ionic downhill movement. The size, charge, length, and tortuosity of the pore are all important determinants of the relative race and extent of diffusion.

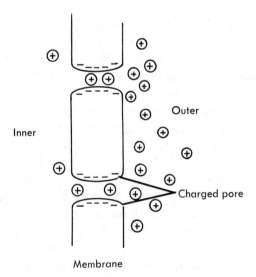

Fig. 1-11. Negatively charged pores of appropriate diameter for sodium movement may be present in membrane.

Several theories speculate that the internal lumen of the pores that are used for ionic movement is either positvely or negatively charged. A postulated scheme for Na^+ diffusion through charged pores is shown in Fig. 1-11. The theoretic pore diameter for the Na^+ pore is 7 Å, and the atomic diameter of a Na^+ ion is 5 Å. The charge and size both act to limit movement through the pores only to Na^+ ions. Separate pores for all diffusible ions are thought to exist.

Diffusion of gases is dependent on the pressure gradient rather than on the concentration gradient per se. Of course, the pressure of a gas in a contained system is dependent on the concentration of gaseous molecules.

Another factor that influences diffusion is the electrochemical gradient of particles that are separated from each other by a membrane. Negatively and positively charged ions obey the laws of electrical attraction and therefore exhibit a tendency to move toward each other. Thus diffusive movement of a charged substance across a membrane would be facilitated by the presence of an oppositely charged membrane interior. Therefore in describing the properties of diffusion one commonly speaks of the *electrochemical gradient*, rather than just the concentration gradient.

Facilitated diffusion

Facilitated diffusion differs from simple diffusion only in one way: the former requires a membrane transport device to move the substance that is diffusing downhill. The rate of facilitated diffusion is therefore limited by the number of available carriers, a phenomenon known as *saturation*. The principle of saturation kinetics is illustrated in Fig. 1-12.

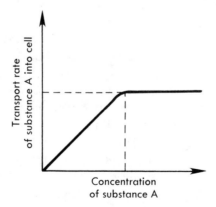

Fig. 1-12. Saturation kinetics are indicated by attainment of maximum rate of transport of substance A, as A increases in concentration. Diagram illustrates saturation of all membrane carriers at certain concentration.

In facilitated diffusion the substance moves downhill only as rapidly as membrane carriers are available to transport it. Some models of facilitated diffusion require that the membrane carrier transport the substance across the membrane and then return to the initial site of uptake to bind with and transport another molecule of the substance. Thus a steep downhill concentration gradient for a substance that moves across a cell membrane might cause an initial rapid diffusion, but as membrane carriers become saturated, the rate of diffusion levels off to a maximum capacity. A later discussion will note that some transportable substances not only require a carrier mechanism but also may require the interaction of another, completely different ion, atom, or molecule before the system can reach maximum activity. Certain cells transport amino acids only in the presence of Na^+ concentration gradient. The Na^+ transport on a carrier that also binds amino acid seems to "drive" the transport of the amino acid. Once Na^+ binds to the carrier, the carrier exhibits an increased affinity for the amino acid.

A physiologically important molecule that enters most cells by facilitated diffusion is glucose. The capacity of the glucose carrier mechanism is probably significantly altered by insulin, which must be present for the diffusion of glucose into many cells. In diabetes mellitus, either there may be no insulin production or there may be cells that are refractory to the insulin that is present. Thus adequate binding of insulin to the cell membrane's insulin receptors does not take place. This binding process appears to be a prerequisite to the next step, which is the diffusion of glucose.

Osmosis

The osmosis of water across a selectively permeable cell membrane can be roughly categorized as a type of diffusion. Osmosis is the diffusion of water across a membrane that restricts the movement of at least one solute. This restriction in solute movement acts to maintain a concentration gradient, even though the solute's tendency is to move downhill. Since the membrane is essentially impermeable to the solute, however, water diffuses down its concentration gradient. The concentration gradient for water is from the less concentrated (more dilute) side of the membrane to the concentrated (less dilute) side. The water will diffuse through exactly the same mechanisms that were previously described for diffusion. Osmosis occurs only if the cell membrane is freely permeable to water. The cell membranes of all human cells are highly permeable to water; thus cells behave like "osmometers," swelling and shrinking in response to the osmotic forces operating on them. The erythrocyte is the best illustration of this phenomenon. When red blood cells are placed in a solution that is very concentrated, such as salty water, the erythrocytes respond through osmosis of water from the interior of the cell to the outside, into the salty water. Shrinkage (crenation) of the cell therefore occurs. When erythrocytes are placed in a solution that contains no salt, such as distilled water, the water will move downhill from the distilled water into the cell, thus swelling the cells. Eventually, after the membranes have been stretched beyond their tolerance, the cells will burst.

A solution that has exactly the same concentrations of osmotically active particles as the cell and ECF is said to be *isotonic* with them. An osmotically active particle is any solute atom, ion, or molecule that is capable of causing osmosis to occur across a membrane in the particular system under question. Thus it is obvious that a substance of a certain weight that contains many small solute particles, as compared to a substance of the same weight that contains large particles, will have a different number of osmotically active particles. The degree to which a solution is osmotically active is measured as *osmotic pressure,* which is the hydrostatic pressure that would be required to totally oppose the osmosis of water from dilute solution into a concentrated one. Osmotic pressure is influenced greatly by the number of osmotically active particles. A solution that is hypotonic to body fluid has a lower osmotic pressure than a hypertonic solution. Osmotic pressure is also dependent on the *activity* of the solute that is separated by the membrane. This colligative property determines the degree to which a solute is dissolved and its true concentration is terms of exerting an osmotic force. Other factors that influence osmotic pressure are seen in the following formula:

$$\pi = \frac{n\,R\,T}{V}$$

In this formula, n is the number of osmotically active particles, π is the osmotic pressure, R is the universal gas constant, T is the absolute temperature, and V is the volume.

A more meaningful term that describes the osmotic activity of solutes is *osmolarity.* If one mole of a substance is present in a solution and does not separate into two or more chemical species, then the osmolarity of the solution is the same as the molarity: *one.* However, if there is dissociation of one mole of a substance into two ions, for example, then one mole of this substance is equal to *two* osmoles. Measurement of the total osmolarity of plasma gives a value of about 300 milliosmoles (mOsm) per liter of plasma fluid. To maintain plasma osmolarity, there must be no net loss or gain of osmotically active solute. Osmolarity can be maintained in a patient receiving IV fluid only if the fluid is isotonic to the plasma. Hypotonic IV fluids will cause a net decrease in the plasma osmolarity initially. The extracellular fluid will gain this fluid as the water osmoses from the bloodstream into the interstitial space. This movement eventually results in a new equilibrium as the plasma and the interstitial fluid reach identical concentrations. However, since there has been a net gain of water, both fluid compartments will have a lower osmotic pressure than that present initially. The reverse is true when an IV infusion of hypertonic substance occurs. Then there will be a net loss of water from the interstitial fluid and a net gain in the plasma. The new osmotic pressure that is reached will be higher than the initial pressure. These changes will occur only if the solute molecules cannot pass through the capillary membranes in significant amounts and thus are able to exert an osmotic pressure. An isotonic dextrose solution (5% dextrose in water) is initially isotonic but becomes hypotonic as the dextrose diffuses across cell membranes and leaves the plasma compartment. Since the glucose is subsequently metabolized within the cells, it also exerts little osmotic pressure there.

The total plasma osmolarity is determined mainly by sodium ions. Albumin, glucose, nitrogenous breakdown products, and other electrolytes make up less than 10% of the osmotic pressure generated by plasma, and the remaining 90% is the result of the Na^+ concentration, which is normally about 144 mEq/liter.

Filtration

Filtration, another important force in maintaining the number and nature of the body fluid compartments, is the process by which fluid moves down its hydrostatic pressure gradient. Gravity is the major determinant of this movement, since hydrostatic pressure is determined by the weight of the fluid. Filtration across a membrane is analogous to filtration of a fluid that is poured through a funnel lined with filter paper. Whatever the filter paper, or membrane, allows to pass will be carried along with the fluid. Filtration is a process that occurs within the capillaries and will be further described in Chapter 2.

Active transport

The phenomena previously discussed (diffusion, osmosis, and filtration) were governed by purely physical laws. The cellular regulation of these processes is determined by the selective permeability of the membrane, but the cell expends no work to cause transport to occur. Thus these transport processes are *passive.*

Active transport implies that metabolic work and energy expenditure must take place. The criteria for active transport include transport against the concentration gradient, saturation kinetics, and metabolic work by the cell. Active transport can be inhibited by cooling the cell, "starving the cell" by not supplying it with glucose, and poisoning the energy-supplying metabolic pathways. Other, more specific "pump" poisons also exist that act on the membrane transport carrier mechanisms. An example is the action of cardiac glycosides, which inhibit the Na^+-K^+ pump. Normally this mechanism pumps out Na^+ and pumps in K^+ against their respective concentration gradients. When a drug such as ouabain or digitalis is present, active transport ceases and the cells accumulate excess sodium and lose potassium.

Normally there is a concentration gradient for Na^+ from outside the cell to inside, causing a tendency for Na^+ to diffuse (or "leak") into the cell. Most cell membranes are relatively impermeable to Na^+, but some Na^+ does leak in over enough time. Eventually an equilibrium would be reached in which the Na^+ concentrations inside and outside the cell were the same. However, this never occurs in the healthy living system. Normally there is about 144 mEq/liter of Na^+ in the ECF and 10 mEq/liter in the ICF. This concentration gradient is maintained through active transport from the cell of all excess Na^+ that leaks into it. Conversely, the high intracellular K^+ concentration is maintained by pumping of K^+ into the cell in a linked manner with active Na^+ efflux. In most cells this transport system involves the release by adenosinetriphosphatase (ATPase), the enzyme that hydrolyzes ATP into adenosine diphosphate (ADP) and phosphate, of free energy that can be coupled to the transport process through the phosphorylation of intermediate molecules. The actual molecular configuration of the Na^+-K^+ pump is not known. The pump is undoubtedly a complex carrier that requires the interaction of the ions that are transported, Ca^{++}, phospholipid, and ATPase. Many other contributing factors have also been identified.

Active transport is utilized for substances other than Na^+ and K^+. A Ca^{++} pump exists in most cells and also plays a major role in muscular contractility. Some amino acids are pumped across cell membranes. An H^+ pump exists in the stomach and kidney tubule, and the secretion of substances into the tubular filtrate often requires active transport.

Larger molecules that cannot diffuse into cells and are not actively transported may move into cells through other energy-expending processes: pinocytosis and phagocytosis. In these mechanisms cells engulf larger molecules, or even bacteria and foreign bodies, in membrane-enclosed vesicles. Cellular energy is of course necessary for this activity. Exocytosis, or extrusion of substances by cells, also requires metabolic work.

SUMMARY

The various fluid compartments are kept separate by the structural and functional integrity of cell membranes.

Transport of solutes and water across these membranes is governed by passive and active processes. Both the selective permeability of a cell membrane and the particular active transport mechanisms of a cell determine the intracellular and extracellular fluids.

The next chapter will examine more closely the compartmental distribution of the body water.

2
Total body water

FLUID COMPARTMENTS

The compartmentalization of the body fluids is accomplished through regulation of the physical and physiologic transport processes described in Chapter 1. The two most all-encompasssing compartments are the intracellular fluid (ICF) and the extracellular fluid (ECF). Within these compartments are subcompartments that are kept structurally and functionally distinct. Table 2-1 delineates the subcompartments of the ECF, which include the blood plasma fluid, the interstitial (tissue) fluid, and the fluid in spaces such as the cerebrospinal fluid, which is contained in the ventricular system of the brain. Other spaces containing small amounts of ECF are the pericardium, the pleura, the peritoneum, and the eyes and ears. Very large amounts of ECF circulate through the entire gastrointestinal tract in every 24-hour period, and at any given time the gut contains 6 to 9 liters of ECF. The total volume of body water (TBW) depends on several factors, such as the age of the individual, the weight, the sex, and the degree of obesity. The standard TBW value, which is for the typical 70 kg adult male, is 60% of the kilogram weight, or 42 to 43 liters of fluid. The ICF is the largest compartment; thus, of the 42 liters of TBW, 32 liters is contained inside cells and the remainder (10 liters) is extracellular. Of the ECF, about 2.5 to 3.0 liters is present as blood plasma, presuming that the hematocrit value is 45% to 50%, since the total blood volume is 5 liters. The remaining ECF is contained mainly within the tissue fluid, and smaller amounts are in the other ECF compartments previously mentioned.

In the newborn the TBW is 80% of the kilogram weight. During the first year of life, which is characterized by rapid growth and increased metabolism, the fluid requirement is 100 ml/kg/24 hr. This is in contrast to the adult requirement of 38 ml/kg/24 hr. The infant's increased demand

Table 2-1. Water compartments

Compartment	TBW (%)
ECF	
Bone, cartilage, connective tissue	15.0
Plasma	7.5
Tissue fluid, lymph	20.0
ICF	55.0
Transcellular	2.5

Table 2-2. Changes in total body water with age

Age	Kilogram weight (%)
Premature infant	80
3 mo	70
6 mo	60
1-2 yr	59
11-16 yr	58
Adult	58-60
Obese adult	40-50
Emaciated adult	70-75

is due to the combination of several contributing factors. A major factor is the proportionately greater ratio of surface area to volume in the infant. Thus proportionately larger amounts of insensible water are lost through the skin. The infant loses 45 ml/kg/24 hr, whereas the adult loss is 15 to 20 ml/kg/24 hr. The threefold greater basal metabolic rate in the infant, with a resultant greater heat production, necessitates a large compartment of insensible water loss, since this is the major mechanism of heat dissipation. Furthermore, because the infant's kidney function is immature, there is a comparative inability to concentrate the urine. Thus a dilute urine having a volume of about 50 ml/kg is produced. With both insensible and urinary losses, the infant's requirements for intake in relation to approximate output are such that an appropriate intake of 100 ml/kg leads to a daily replacement of one third of the infant's ECF. The further implication is that the infant's entire ECF compartment is replaced (turned over) every 3 days!

It is necessary to point out here that although the amount of fluid contained within each of these compartments is relatively constant, there is nevertheless a continuous exchange of both solutes and water between them. Thus there is a dynamic exchange that functions to constantly maintain the specific characteristics of each compartment.

The percentage of TBW decreases with age, the highest percentage of water per kilogram being present in the infant and the lowest in the elderly person. Table 2-2 shows the various percentages that occur throughout the life cycle.

The degree of obesity present in an individual is another important determinant of TBW. Adipose tissue contains large amounts of lipid stored within the cells, or adipocytes. Although the total number of adipocytes is probably attained by the first year of life, there can be variable amounts of lipid stored within these cells throughout life. In obesity, increased amounts of lipid are contained within the adipose tissue. Lipid is hydrophobic, and therefore adipose tissue contains very little cellular water. Since more of the kilogram weight is present as adipose tissue, there will be less TBW. Water deficit may develop rapidly in an obese person who loses water through such water loss machanisms as sweating, fever, diarrhea, or vomiting. Women have less TBW than men in proportion to their weight, primarily because of their greater fat reserves.

The TBW is maintained in health through a balance of water intake and output. If excess fluid is lost, compensatory mechanisms are activated to increase intake. If a primary increase in TBW occurs, then the excess will be excreted or lost as a result of compensation.

Water intake is achieved through either drinking or eating, and of course water is metabolically produced through oxidative metabolism (300 ml/24 hr). Output, however, can take place through several routes, namely the urine, the feces, the skin, and the lungs. Regulation of intake is basically through the thirst mechanism; output is regulated by a variety of control measures.

Thirst mechanism

The desire for water and the accompanying behavior that causes an animal to search for water are neurologically integrated and regulated. The center for thirst control lies in specific neurons in the hypothalamus. Fig. 2-1 diagrams the control of thirst. The major stimulants of the hypothalamic thirst center are increased plasma osmolarity and decreased blood volume. Thirst is also affected by corticohypothalamic impulses, and psychologic factors therefore may play a role. Mucous membrane dehydration leading to the sensation of a "dry throat" also leads to a feeling of thirst.

The thirst center cells of the hypothalamus are considered to be *osmo-*

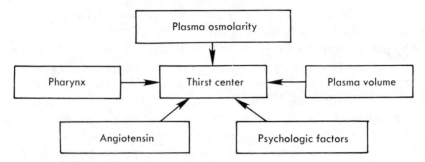

Fig. 2-1. Thirst is regulated through plasma osmolarity and volume. Receptors in pharynx also may supply information to hypothalamic thirst center.

receptors, which osmotically shrink or swell in response to plasma osmotic pressure. When water in excess of electrolytes is lost, the plasma becomes hypertonic. The cells of the hypothalamus shrink as cytoplasmic water osmoses into the plasma, and the result is an activation of thirst sensation and water-seeking behavior. The converse process occurs if the plasma is hypotonic: the cells swell and the absence of thirst results.

Volume receptors that have direct input into the thirst center are believed to exist as well, since it is known that thirst is activated by a loss of overall plasma volume without an accompanying change in plasma osmolarity. For example, people who have suffered an extensive loss of blood (hemorrhage) experience a profound thirst sensation. Volume receptors that send messages to the thirst center may be present in the right atrium and venae cavae.

Angiotensin II is a chemical mediator that forms in the blood when the kidneys release renin. Renin is released in response to a decrease in blood volume. The angiotensin II, although only transiently present, nevertheless has several important effects: it stimulates the secretion of antidiuretic hormone (ADH), increases gut water reabsorption, and stimulates neurons near the thirst center, which then send input into the thirst center, activating thirst sensation. However, recent evidence summarized by Stricker suggests that angiotensin-driven thirst plays a minor role in the overall thirst mechanism.

Thirst, although a necessary survival drive, is not accurately regulated in the human. Thus humans never respond to water loss with the exact water intake needed to repair the loss. Other regulatory mechanisms must be called into play to accomplish the "fine tuning" of water balance.

Another important factor in water balance is that the thirst center requires an alert state in the individual. Infants, persons with cerebro-cortical depression or in coma, psychologically disturbed persons, and some aged persons are unable to respond appropriately to the sensation of thirst. Although the actual sensation may be perceived, the appropriate behavioral responses may not be sufficiently integrated or, in the case of the infant, may not be mature. Thus persons in these groups are at risk for the rapid development of dehydration if proper early assessment and intervention are not carried out.

Hormonal control of water balance

Antidiuretic hormone. Whereas thirst controls water intake, several other mechanisms act to control output when water deprivation occurs. Obviously, when water deficit is present, the urinary loss must decrease to preserve the plasma volume. The major regulator of urinary water loss is ADH. This hormone is released by the neurohypophysis (posterior pituitary gland) in response to decreased blood volume or increased plasma osmolarity. ADH is actually synthesized by cells in the supraoptic and paraventricular nuclei in the hypothalamus, transported down neurons into the neurohypophysis, and stored there until needed by the body. ADH influences blood pressure elevation and, most importantly, water retention through its action on the collecting duct of certain nephrons in the kidneys. This hormone is continuously released, but the amounts increase when the plasma osmolarity increases or the plasma volume drops. The possibility exists that the same neurons involved in thirst also control ADH secretion, since the stimuli for both are the same. Osmo-receptors that activate ADH release and that also act on thirst are questioned by some. Sodium-sensitive receptors appear to be present in the area around the ventricles in the brain. Infusion of solutions containing differing amounts of sodium into the cerebrospinal fluid results in the expected alterations in thirst and ADH secretion. However, sucrose solutions of varying osmotic strengths do not at all cause the expected responses, based on the osmoreceptor theory (Anderson).

ADH acts to decrease urine output and increase water conservation by altering the water permeability of the cells of the renal collecting ducts. Under the influence of ADH, these cells become freely permeable to water, and because of the osmotic pressure of the interstitial fluid, water leaves the fluid of the collecting ducts and osmoses into the interstitium and from there into the plasma. The mode of action of ADH is not known. Tubular cells apparently bind molecules of the hormone, a phenomenon that results in subsequent activation of the adenyl cyclase system. Cyclic adenosine monophosphate (cAMP) is then released into the cytoplasm. The usual action of cAMP is to effect a protein kinase system that activates a previously inactive enzyme or protein. The specific activated protein in tubular cells has not been identified, but the effect of cAMP increase is ultimately to increase cellular permeability to water. Perhaps water pores that are normally closed become open in the presence of ADH.

ADH secretion also occurs in response to stress and may be prolonged. The result of surgical stress is often several days of fluid retention caused by ADH excess. Some drugs (e.g., morphine) increase ADH release, whereas ethanol significantly depresses it, thus accounting for the diuresis that follows ingestion of excess alcohol.

One other hormone, oxytocin, is released from the neurohypophysis. It is important in initiating uterine contractions during the three stages of labor and in causing the ejection of milk from the breast in lactating women. Previously, posterior pituitary extracts containing oxytocin (Pitocin) were administered intravenously to women for the purpose of inducing labor. Such preparations also contained ADH, however, and an occasionally severe and often prolonged antidiuretic effect was seen in these women. Oxytocin extracts today are much freer of ADH activity, but the amino acid composition of these two hormones is extremely similar, and fluid assessment of the woman whose labor is being induced is of great importance.

Aldosterone. Another hormonally mediated control of the TBW involves the secretion of aldosterone from the adrenal cortex. This hormone also acts on the renal tubular epithelium, primarily at the distal convoluted tubule, and regulates *facilitory* water reabsorption by acting to increase sodium uptake from the tubular fluid, through the renal interstitium, and thence to the plasma. This amount of water retention is known as facilitory because it occurs only in response to the sodium reabsorption and is osmotic in nature. Water reabsorption in the kidney that is *obligatory* occurs as the osmotic accompaniment of solute reabsorption that cannot be altered. A certain amount of solute reabsorption proceeds inevitably, particularly in the proximal tubule, and water follows it osmotically without physiologic regulation or alteration. Aldosterone, for example, has no effect on water and sodium reabsorption in the proximal tubule, where most of the total sodium uptake occurs.

The aldosterone release mechanism will be discussed in more detail in Chapters 4 and 7. Here it is mentioned only to indicate that water loss routes such as the kidneys are carefully regulated through hormonal mechanisms. The major stimulus to aldosterone release is decreased plasma volume, which is sensed by specialized renal cells that respond by releasing the substance *renin*. A variety of biochemical mediators are produced in the blood as the result of renin release, and the final result is stimulation of the adrenal cortex to release aldosterone.

Organs of water loss

The organs of water loss are the kidneys, skin, lungs, and gastrointestinal tract.

Kidneys. To summarize general aspects of renal regulation of water loss, the following should be noted: Although the kidneys normally filter 170 liters of plasma per day, only 1.5 liters of urine is excreted. The major regulation of fluid balance is through the kidneys. Several processes are regulated, including the amount and rate of glomerular filtration, the extent of solute reabsorption, and the degree of water permeability.

The urine must consist of an adequate volume to dilute the wastes that must be excreted daily. The range of concentrating ability, which is from 50 to 1400 mOsm/liter, is analogous to a specific gravity range of 1.001 to 1.040. A normal diet of 3000 kcal produces 1200 mOsm, an amount that is well within the ability of the kidney to excrete without excessive water loss. An individual with renal disease or an infant may have difficulty concentrating the urine, however, and thus the excretion of 1200 mOsm through the kidneys could result in excessive water loss if, for example, the kidneys were not able to concentrate the urine above 600 mOsm/liter. In this case 2 liters of fluid would be lost as dilute urine.

The kidneys' role in fluid, electrolyte, acid, and base balance will be further described in Chapter 4.

Skin. Regulation of water loss from the skin is mainly through the sympathetic nervous system (SNS), which innervates the sweat glands. These glands are also affected to a minor degree by aldosterone.

SNS stimulation of the sweat glands causes them to increase sweat production. Sweating is an effective way for excess heat produced internally to be released into the external environment. In muscular exercise, for example, large amounts of heat are produced. The core temperature elevates, but dangerous levels of heat are shunted off through perspiration.

Water loss from the skin has both *sensible* and *insensible* components. Insensible water loss occurs continuously from the skin and lungs and is evaporative. It is not perceived by the individual in any way, but in a young adult 15 to 20 ml/kg/24 hr is regularly lost by this route. With this amount of water loss, 972 kcal of heat energy is also dissipated, since 0.58 kcal is utilized for every milliliter of insensible water loss. Insensible water loss is greatly affected by body temperature. For every degree Celsius of fever in an individual, a 10% increase in insensible water loss occurs. This loss very often accounts for most of the dehydration that occurs with high fever but is nevertheless insensible and must be separated from sensible sweating, which is perceived as moisture on the skin. Sensible loss in the normal adult ranges from 0 to 5000 ml/24 hr, depending on amount of exercise and ambient temperature, beginning when the temperature exceeds (27° C) (80° F). Without this mechanism the option of temperature regulation, a characteristic of endothermic, or warm-blooded, animals, would not be possible. Warm-blooded animals either pant or sweat and thus can maintain their core body temperature at the normal set point through evaporative heat dissipation. Of course, other mechanisms must come into play when a living organism loses extracellular water through sensible perspiration. Behavioral responses are required; that is, the animal must seek the cool of the shade and must find and drink appropriate amounts of water to replace the loss. Regulatory and compensatory physiologic controls are also activated; for example, the urine of a sweating individual becomes more concentrated and smaller in volume. Evolutionary factors play a role as well. The desert mammal is able to make a much more concentrated urine and thus loses less water than mammals in cooler environments.

The composition of insensible and sensible perspiration is different. Both fluids are, however, *hypotonic* to plasma. Insensible water loss is basically electrolyte and solute free—in other words, the fluid lost is nearly pure water. Sensible perspiration contains some sodium, potassium, and other electrolytes. However, it is a common misconception to consider sensible sweat as *hypertonic* because it tastes salty. The salty taste is caused by the evaporation of the water in the sweat, which of course leaves behind the solute. Thus the sweat on the skin surface becomes hypertonic as the water evaporates.

The maximum water loss through sweat is 2 liters/hr, but without water and solute replacement this rate could not be maintained very long! A requirement of heat loss through sensible sweating is the presence of a vapor tension gradient from the skin to the air so that the sweat can evaporate. Thus heat dissipation by sweating is not effective on hot, humid days. Furthermore there is a limit to the rate at which the body can dissipate heat, even when sweating is maximal. If excessive heat is produced and not dissipated, a time is reached when the central hypo-thalamic mechanisms for heat loss and gain become impaired. Sweating can then no longer occur, and the result is a dangerous progression of in-creasingly higher temperatures.

Lungs. Insensible water loss occurs at approximate daily rates of 600 to 800 ml through skin and an additional 400 ml through the lungs (expired air is saturated at 35° C). Losses may increase in this compart-ment (the lungs) as a result of increased respiratory rate or depth or both. The administration of dry oxygen can also lead to water loss through the respiratory tract, as can the use of a ventilator for an extended period.

Gastrointestinal tract. The gastrointestinal tract constitutes a fluid compartment that maintains a large circulation of fluid—as much as 7 liters/24 hr. However, the usual fecal water loss is only 100 ml/24 hr. Water that is taken into the gut through food and fluid ingestion is ab-sorbed into ECF mainly through the walls of the small intestine. Mixed with this fluid is the fluid output of the stomach, pancreas, gallbladder, and intestinal glands. The regulation of secretion of the gut fluids is largely hormonal and neural. Reabsorption occurs through diffusive, osmotic, and active transport processes and is mediated also through hormonal mechanisms such as ADH.

Summary of water gain and loss

Water gain is basically regulated through the thirst drive. Water loss is even more carefully controlled through the kidneys, skin, sweat, lungs, and gastrointestinal tract. The aim of intake and output regulation is to maintain a balance so that the TBW remains constant. Furthermore the internal constancy, which is present in spite of dynamic flux, is controlled. Water balance is the result of a complex interaction of many sensing mechanisms and regulatory processes.

So far we have described only water compartments. There is no pure water compartment, except perhaps for insensible water. All other fluid compartments contain varying concentrations of particular solutes. Thus water loss from the ECF may also cause solute loss if, for example, ECF is lost into a burn. Water from the ECF without accompanying solute may also occur if water osmoses from the ECF into the ICF.

• • •

The following section describes normal electrolyte balance. Electrolyte disturbances and their pathophysiologic effects will be discussed in subse-quent chapters.

ELECTROLYTE COMPARTMENTS

The major difference in electrolyte concentrations in both the intracellular and extracellular compartments is the distribution of Na^+ and K^+. The K^+ ion is the major intracellular cation. A cation is a positively charged ion, and within the body fluids there is a net balance of cations and anions (negatively charged ions). Ions are electrolytes, which means that when a negative cathode and a positive anode are placed in an electrolyte-containing fluid, there is a migration of anions to the anode and of cations to the cathode. This implies, further, that an electrolyte solution can carry an electrical charge, as illustrated in Fig. 2-2. Certain chemical substances naturally *ionize*, or split into ions, when they are placed in a solvent. Strong acids ionize more freely than weak acids, and it is the hydrogen ion that is produced which gives acids their caustic quality. The same is true for strong bases; their "strength" is a measure of their degree of ionization. The hydroxyl ion determines the caustic properties of a strong base. Salts ionize in solution as well. When NaCl crystals are placed in water (the solvent), there is an instantaneous and total dissociation of the molecule into Na^+ and Cl^- ions. There is net neutrality of the solutions because equal and equivalent negative and positive charges are

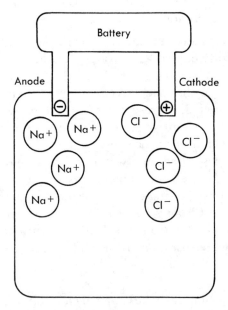

Fig. 2-2. Anions (Cl^-) migrate to cathode and cations (Na^+) to anode in solution of NaCl.

present. One could, however, remove all the Na⁺ from the solution by creating a current of Na⁺ toward a cathode. Thus we can see that electrolyte solutions are capable of conducting an electrical current.

The ionic constituents of electrolyte solutions are measured in *milliequivalents* rather than in standard weights such as milligrams or millimoles (mmole).

Table 2-3 lists the various ways that substances are measured chemically and defines the units of measurement. It can be seen that a milliequivalent is a measure of the electrical equivalency of a substance. If a millimole of an electrolyte that is divalent (has two positive or negative charges) is measured in milliequivalents, then 1 mmole of the substance is equal to 2 mEq, because of the two charges on the ion. One millimole of a trivalent ion is equal to 3 mEq. A mole is the gram molecular weight (and a millimole is one one-thousandth of a mole), a value equal to Avogadro's number (6.02×10^{23} particles in a mole). The term *mole*

Table 2-3. Common units of electrolyte measurement

Unit of measurement	Definition
Millimole (mmole): 0.001 mole	Atomic or molecular weight of a substance in milligrams (mg). For example, since the molecular weight of sodium is 23, 1 mmole Na = 23 mg.
Milliequivalent (mEq): 0.001 equivalent	Amount of substance in milligrams (mg) that can combine or replace 1 mg hydrogen (since atomic weight of hydrogen is 1). Examples:
	Sodium:
	1 mmole Na⁺ = 23 mg Valence of Na⁺ = 1 1 mEq Na⁺ = 1 mmole 1 mmole Na⁺ = 23 mg 1 mEq = 23 mg
	Calcium:
	1 mmole Ca⁺⁺ = 40 mg (atomic weight = 40) Valence of Ca⁺⁺ = 2 1 mmole Ca⁺⁺ = 2 mEq 2 mEq Ca⁺⁺ = 40 × 2 = 80 mg
Milliosmole (mOsm): 0.001 osmole)	Unit of osmolarity (related to number of osmotically active particles in the solution). For substances that do not ionize, 1 mmole = 1 mOsm. If substance ionizes into two particles, 1 mmole = 2 mOsm. Example: NaCl → Na⁺ + Cl⁻ 1 mmole NaCl = 2 mOsm

Table 2-4. Normal concentrations and functions of the major body electrolytes*

Electrolyte	Serum concentration (in plasma)	Functions
Sodium (Na)	137-142 mEq/liter	Retention of fluid in body Generation and transmission of nerve impulses Maintenance of acid-base balance Replacement of potassium in cell Enzyme activities Regulation of osmolarity and electroneutrality of cell
Potassium (K)	3.4-4.5 mEq/liter	Maintenance of regular cardiac rhythm Deposition of glycogen in liver cells Function of enzyme systems necessary for cell energy production Transmission and conduction of nerve impulses Regulation of osmolarity and electroneutrality of cell
Calcium (Ca)	5 mEq/liter	Formation of bone and teeth (calcium phosphate) Transmission of nerve impulse Muscular contraction Clotting of blood Maintenance of cell membrane permeability
Chloride (Cl)	97-103 mEq/liter	Transport of CO_2 (chloride shift) Formation of hydrochloric acid in stomach Retention of potassium Maintenance of osmolarity of cell

*From Groër, M. E., and Shekleton, M. E.: Basic pathophysiology: a conceptual approach, St. Louis, 1979, The C. V. Mosby Co.

gives no information about charge, but the term *milliequivalent,* on the other hand, is used only for charged substances. In physiology, rather than speaking of absolute amounts of electrolytes in body fluids, the *concentration* of the ions in milliequivalents per liter is commonly described. Table 2-4 shows these concentration values for the important intracellular and extracellular ions.

It is possible to measure the amounts of different solutes contained within the body water compartments. Radioactive solutes of known amount and concentration are injected into experimental animals whose volumes of TBW, ECF, and ICF are known. Dilution of the injected radioactivity is then measured, and a close approximation of the true concentrations of the "cold" (nonradioactive) solute can be determined. With this method, not only can the amounts of solute be measured, but the presence of nonexchangeable compartments of various solutes is also cal-culated. Such sequestered solute compartments may have great im-portance in estimations of excesses or deficits.

There are major differences between intracellular and extracellular solute concentrations; yet it is important to note that the sums of the cations and anions in both compartments are the same. Both compart-ments are electrically neutral.

The concentrations of the solutes are maintained through the perme-ability properties of cell membranes and the activity of linked Na^+-K^+ pumping. Another contribution is made by plasma protein, which is nega-tively charged and which also occupies a certain volume of each milli-liter of plasma. Thus the *plasma* concentrations of various substances are technically inaccurate and should be corrected *for* protein-occupying volume. The Na^+ value of 142 mEq/liter in plasma is in reality 153 mEq/liter of plasma *water*.

Table 2-4 shows the functions of the major body electrolytes. It should be stressed that not only the normal concentrations of these substances but also their compartmental distribution must be maintained. It is im-portant to emphasize that the concentration value may change drastically even though there is no change in the total body amount. For example, if a water loss or gain occurred in the ECF, there would be resultant con-centration or dilution effects on any solutes present in the ECF. If water in excess of solute is lost from the ECF, there will be a resultant increase in the concentration of contained solutes and any other particles, such as platelets, white blood cells, and erythrocytes. Addition of excess solute-free water would have a converse dilutive effect. For most electrolyte ef-fects on physiological function, it is the *concentration* of the electrolyte rather than the absolute amount that is essential.

CAPILLARY DYNAMICS

If the electrolytes of the various body compartments are to remain at equilibrium concentrations, the fluid movements across the membranes that separate fluid compartments must not disrupt this balance. Fluid movement from the plasma into the interstitial fluid occurs at the capil-laries, which are diffusely distributed throughout all the body tissues. Thus the major barrier separating these two components of the ECF is the thin-walled capillary membrane, which is made up of loosely adja-cent *endothelial cells*. Capillaries arise from the multiple branching of the arterioles as they supply the various body tissues (Fig. 2-3) and con-

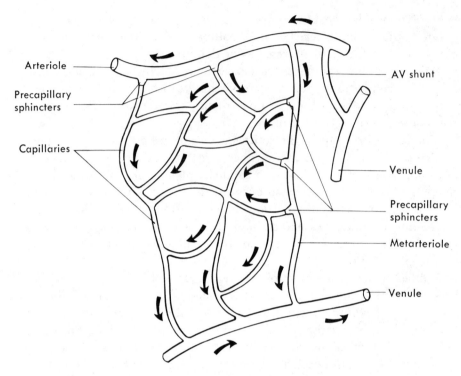

Fig. 2-3. Microcirculation. (From Groër, M. E., and Shekleton, M. E.: Basic pathophysiology: a conceptual approach, St. Louis, 1979, The C. V. Mosby Co.)

verge to form venules, which then carry the now deoxygenated blood to the right side of the heart. Essentially all of the cardiac output (5 liters/min) moves through the capillaries, which are able to withstand the volume and pressure of the blood because of their small size. Capillaries can hold this blood without significant changes in wall tension, since, according to Laplace's law:

$$T \propto P \times R$$

where T = tension, P = pressure, and R = radius. As the radius of a vessel decreases, at a constant pressure, the wall tension also proportionately decreases. Capillary radius does not change, but blood flow and pressure through the capillaries are altered by the size of the arterioles and precapillary sphincters. These are innervated by the sympathetic nervous system and are the sites of the major resistance to blood flow that occurs in the vascular tree. With constriction of the arteriole and sphincter, the blood flowing from the heart meets a resistance to flow, which essentially makes it more difficult for the blood to flow through the capillaries. If the blood flow through the capillaries is to be maintained when the arterioles are constricted, there must be a greater pressure applied to the blood as it is ejected from the heart. This general phenomenon is described by the following formula:

$$\dot{Q} = \Delta P/R$$

where $\dot{Q}$ = flow, ΔP = change in pressure, and R = resistance. This formula should be memorized because it will be useful in the study of both cardiovascular dynamics and fluid flow dynamics.

The preceding discussion implies that blood circulates through the capillaries at the rate of 5 liters/min. Certain tissue beds receive more of the cardiac output than others, depending on metabolic demand and size of the tissue bed. The amount of blood delivered to a capillary bed depends on whether there are open, relaxed arterioles and precapillary sphincters through which blood ejected during cardiac systole can easily flow. Thus the state of sympathetic nervous system activity in a given capillary bed is of great importance in determining the flow through it. Since alternate constriction and relaxation of the precapillary vessels are present in any capillary bed, the flow through the individual capillaries is variable. This phenomenon is called *vasomotion*. Another, equally great influence on capillary flow is the metabolic needs of the tissue supplied by the capillary bed. Through the property of autoregulation, arterioles and precapillary sphincters open and close under the influence of various tissue metabolites. An active tissue will utilize oxygen, produce carbon dioxide, and release other products of metabolism such as adenosine and lactic acid. It is believed that accumulation of these substances in the tissue fluids acts directly to dilate the resistance vessels, causing an increased flow of blood through the capillaries. It will be seen that this increased amount of blood results in greater oxygenation of the tissue, as well as an increase in the supply of nutrients to the tissue and the washing out of the waste products from the capillary bed.

• • •

The next section will describe in detail the process of filtration and reabsorption of fluid through the capillaries, as well as the general mechanisms by which transport of nutrients and waste products move through the capillary endothelium.

Capillary endothelium

Basic to a discussion of the body fluids is an understanding of the morphologic and functional nature of the capillary endothelium. This tissue rings the capillaries and forms a loose lining permeable to most of the dissolved substances in the blood plasma. Recall that the capillary membrane must be highly permeable to allow the rapid movement of fluid and solutes to and from plasma and interstitial fluid. Furthermore this membrane must allow the fluid balance between these two compartments to be maintained. How does the capillary membrane permit the diffusion of substances across it and also allow the tremendous flow of fluid back and forth across it? There are two possible explanations for these phenomena, as seen in Fig. 2-4. Some have suggested that vesicles formed at the endothelial surface act as transporters of substances from one side to the other. Electron micrographs of capillary endothelial cells show vesicles that appear to be able to move through the cell. Another mode of

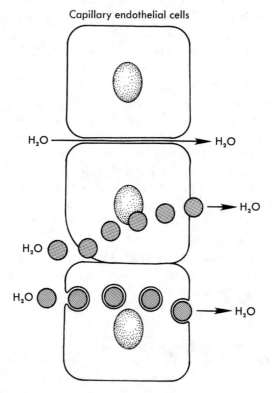

Fig. 2-4. Water movement across capillary endothelium may occur through gaps between cells or via vesicles moving across cells.

transport, certainly more plausible for water movement, involves the spaces between the adjacent endothelial cells. These spaces range from 100 to 200 Angstrom units (Å) in width. The fluid movement through the capillaries seems to take place primarily through these intercellular spaces.

Of course, some molecules are able to diffuse directly through the cells themselves. We tend to lose sight of the importance of simple diffusion as we study the mechanics of fluid flow across the capillary membrane. In actuality, diffusion is the most important way by which molecules move through the endothelium. Gases such as oxygen and carbon dioxide, for example, diffuse readily and rapidly through the cells of the endothelium. Many solute molecules also diffuse well. Diffusion is 5000 times more rapid than filtration and reabsorption of fluid across the capillary bed. The latter two processes allow a flow of fluid to wash through the tissue spaces constantly. There is an actual circulation of plasma fluid through the capillary endothelium from the arterial end of the capillary, thence to the interstitial space, and then back again into the venous end of the capillary. Of course, there is water and solute movement all along the length of the capillary, and there is no net loss or gain of fluid into the interstitial space as the result of this circulation. The basic nature of this circulation was first described by Starling, and Starling's law of the capillaries described the mechanisms involved.

Starling's law of the capillaries

The blood that enters the capillaries does so at a certain pressure, called the blood hydrostatic pressure. This pressure of the capillary fluid is imparted to the fluid as the result of (1) the dynamic ejection of the fluid from the heart and (2) the actual force of gravity (weight) acting on the blood. Therefore, since hydrostatic pressure is basically caused by gravity, some capillary beds will have a much higher capillary pressure merely because of their location. The capillary beds in the feet, for example, are subjected to much higher hydrostatic pressures than the capillaries of the hands.

The average blood hydrostatic pressure, as it enters the capillaries, is 32 mm Hg. This pressure is exerted in an outward direction from the capillary blood onto the capillary walls. It is therefore a filtration force, and since the capillary membrane is so highly permeable to fluid, there will be a movement of fluid from the capillary into the tissue spaces. Of course, there may be some opposition to this outward filtering force if the tissue fluid itself exerts some hydrostatic pressure against this filtering force.

There is controversy about the nature of the tissue pressure. Some physiologists believe that there is an actual negative pressure, or vacuum, in the tissue spaces, and this would cause the tissue fluid to exert a sucking inward force on the fluid contained in the capillary. Others believe that a positive tissue fluid pressure of approximately 1 or 2 mm Hg is present in most capillary beds. Thus, to determine the net filtering force at the arterial end, it is necessary to know both the blood hydrostatic pressure and the tissue hydrostatic pressure. If the blood hydrostatic pressure is +21 mm Hg, and the tissue pressure is −6 mm Hg, then the total outward force is 38 mm Hg, since the vacuum provided by the interstitium is additive with the filtering-out force:

$$32 - (-6) = 32 + 6 = 38$$

On the other hand, an interstitial fluid pressure of +2 mm Hg would oppose fluid movement and must therefore be subtracted from the hydrostatic fluid force of the capillary blood. In this case, then, the net outward force would be 32 − 2, or 30 mm Hg.

As the fluid filters out of the capillary, its pressure gradually drops along the capillary length. Another important force must therefore be considered in accounting for the fact that no net loss or gain of fluid occurs in any given capillary bed. This force is osmotic in nature and is due to the following facts: First, the capillary membrane is selectively permeable, and although it permits most dissolved substances to cross it, it is only slightly permeable to proteins. Thus protein is kept contained within the capillary fluid as fluid filters out into the interstitial space. Since the protein is so contained, it exerts an osmotic pressure, which is known as the *oncotic* or *colloid osmotic* pressure. Albumin is largely responsible for this pressure because it is the smallest blood protein, and therefore the many albumin molecules exert an osmotic force on the interstitial fluid, causing it to move osmotically into the capillary. Second, the interstitial fluid offers some osmotic pressure of its own, and it opposes the plasma colloid osmotic pressure. The reason is that small amounts of protein do, with time, leak out of the plasma into the tissue space. These proteins cannot move back into the plasma and thus are osmotically active, causing water to move from the plasma into the interstitium in an osmotic manner. A significant accumulation of protein in the interstitial fluid is therefore theoretically possible with time, but this is prevented by the operation of the lymphatic system, which acts to drain excessive fluid and protein that might otherwise be present. Lymphatic capillaries are highly permeable blind pouches that form lymphatic vessels. Eventually the lymphatic vessels converge and empty into the

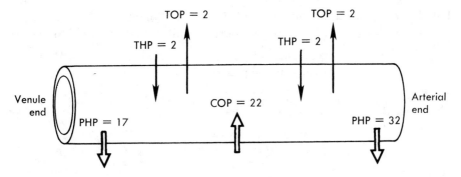

Fig. 2-5. Capillary pressures and tissue pressures determine net filtration and reabsorption of fluid. *TOP* = tissue osmotic pressure; *THP* = tissue hydrostatic pressure; *COP* = colloid osmotic pressure; *PHP* = plasma hydrostatic pressure.

venous circulation, thus returning the fluid and protein into the bloodstream. Additionally, the lymphatic nodes that are present along the length of the vessels screen the lymph fluid and thus act as an important body defense.

Colloid osmotic pressure remains fairly constant along the length of the capillary. A typical value for this pressure is 22 mm Hg, and the tissue osmotic pressure is about 2 mm Hg. Therefore the total inward osmotic force would be 22 − 2, or 20 mm Hg.

Following the forces that affect fluid movement along the length of the capillary, it can be seen in Fig. 2-5 that only one force changes significantly from the arterial to the venule end of the capillary: the hydrostatic pressure of the capillary blood. This pressure drops from 32 mm Hg at the arterial end to 17 mm Hg at the venous end. All other forces remaining constant, the outward forces at the arterial end of the capillary are:

Plasma hydrostatic pressure	32
Tissue osmotic pressure	+ 2
	34

The inward forces here are:

Colloid osmotic pressure	22
Tissue hydrostatic pressure	+ 2
	24

Therefore the total force is:

$$34 - 24 = 10 \text{ mm Hg outward pressure}$$

This force causes a *net* filtration of fluid at the arterial end of the capillary. Conversely, at the venous end of the capillary the outward forces are:

Plasma hydrostatic pressure	17
Tissue osmotic pressure	+ 2
	19

The inward forces here are:

Colloid osmotic pressure	22
Tissue hydrostatic pressure	+ 2
	24

Therefore the total force is:

$$24 - 19 = 5 \text{ mm Hg inward pressure}$$

This force causes net reabsorption of fluid into the venous end of the capillary. It is important to note that in this example the pressure driving fluid out of the arterial end and thus the fluid amount driven out are not completely balanced by the inward pressures and fluid movement at the venule end. Thus a circulation of fluid through the capillary bed occurs, causing a slight loss of fluid. The fluid lost into the tissue spaces is returned to the blood by the lymphatic system at the rate of 2 to 4 liters/24 hr.

Many pathologic conditions can alter the normal filtration and reabsorption forces at the capillary level. Changes in hydrostatic pressure, osmotic forces, and capillary integrity will all have major influences on the Starling mechanisms. The first example with clinical relevance is the fluid dynamics that can take place in dehydration: Since less fluid will be contained within the cardiovascular system, the hydrostatic pressure of the remaining fluid will be lower than normal. Furthermore, since osmotic pressure is the result of the *concentration* of osmotically active particles, the fluid loss will cause an increased colloid osmotic pressure. Both of these forces will now act at the capillary level to cause less filtration out of, and increased reabsorption into, the capillary fluid. It can be seen that this adaptive function allows the dehydrated person to experience an "autotransfusion" of tissue fluid into the dehydrated vascular system. Of course, overhydration has the exact opposite effect, resulting in a net increase in filtration out of the capillary fluid and into the tissue fluid. When excess fluid begins to accumulate in the tissue spaces, *edema* develops.

Second, another alteration in net fluid forces at the capillary level occurs when the plasma proteins are decreased. In starvation, for example, hypoalbuminemia develops, causing a drop in the plasma oncotic pressure. Therefore a major reabsorption force is decreased, and the resultant net filtration into the tissue spaces causes edema. Photographs of children suffering from severe calorie-protein malnutrition may portray a falsely healthy picture because of their swollen faces and abdomens. This swelling is the result of decreased colloid osmotic pressure and resultant tissue edema.

A third example of disruption of capillary fluid forces is seen in patients with severe traumatic injuries or burns. When the capillary endothelium is traumatized, it becomes highly permeable, and the result is leakage of plasma proteins into the interstitial fluid. The fluid and protein accumulate there, with a loss of Starling forces, since essentially either no barrier or only a slight one now exists between the plasma and tissue fluid. The burned patient can become extremely dehydrated in terms of the vascular fluid compartment, since so much plasma fluid and protein may be lost into the burn wound because of the increased capillary membrane permeability.

Subsequent chapters will discuss in greater detail the clinical conditions that have been described.

SUMMARY

This chapter has emphasized the distribution of water and electrolytes into various compartments and the regulation of TBW as well as water and electrolyte compartments. Mechanisms of importance include thirst, hormonal control, and sensible and insensible loss through the kidneys, skin, lungs, and gastrointestinal tract. Electrolyte distributions and the regulation of their specific concentrations by the above mechanisms have been also included, and the capillary dynamics that control the movement of plasma and interstitial fluid have been discussed.

Chapter 3 will elaborate on the role of electrolytes in the maintenance of the cell membrane potential and in excitability.

3

Physiology of the cell membrane

This chapter will present the normal electrophysiology of the cell membrane. Considerable detail is included because a good foundation in this topic helps in understanding the effects of electrolyte alteration. Although it is possible to simply memorize the signs and symptoms of electrolyte deficiencies and excesses, it will be much easier to recall them in clinical settings if the basic cell disruptions are understood.

GIBBS-DONNAN RELATIONSHIP

Before the origin of the resting membrane potential is described, it is necessary to discuss the reason for the peculiar distribution of ions across a cell membrane. This distribution is partly due to the Gibbs-Donnan relationship, which is caused by the impermeability of the cell membrane to most intracellular anions, including negatively charged proteins. Recall that simple solutions of ions are at electrical equilibrium, the result of a balance of anions and cations. However, in cells, since some of the cell anions are not free to move out of the cell, those smaller anions that can move are driven out and therefore have a lower intracellular concentration than would be expected. The nondiffusible intracellular anion causes more diffusible cation to be intracellular and more diffusible anion to be extracellular. The net result is shown in the following relationship:

$$K^+ \text{ (inside)} > K^+ \text{ (outside)}$$
$$Cl^- \text{ (inside)} < Cl^- \text{ (outside)}$$

and:

$$\frac{K^+ \text{ (inside)}}{K^+ \text{ (outside)}} = \frac{Cl^- \text{ (outside)}}{Cl^- \text{ (inside)}}$$

Since intracellular protein does not diffuse, the intracellular compartment has more solute particles than the extracellular one and therefore exerts a greater osmotic pressure:

$$K^+ \text{ (inside)} + Cl^- \text{ (inside)} + Prot^- \text{ (inside)} > K^+ \text{ (outside)} Cl^- \text{ (outside)}$$

Furthermore, the sum of the anions not being equal to the sum of the cations, there is an excess of anions on the inside and an excess of cations on the outside. The result is a very slight charge difference between the cell fluid and the extracellular fluid (ECF) that contributes, as we shall see, to the membrane potential. In addition, the Gibbs-Donnan relationship predicts that cells have a tendency to swell osmotically and in fact would do so to the point of rupture (lysis) if the cell's ionic active transport machinery were inoperative. The assumption is that K^+ and Cl^- are the major diffusible ions across cell membranes. If Na^+ should suddenly enter a cell, the Gibbs-Donnan relationship would be disrupted. The cell therefore maintains a relative impermeability to Na^+ by actively extruding any excess Na^+ greater than the steady-state level that leaks into the cell.

Another important point to consider is the response of the cell to ionic changes in the ECF. If, for example, the Cl^- concentration in the ECF dropped drastically, there would be less anion in the ECF, and K^+ and Cl^- would move out of the cell to balance the loss so that the following relationship would be maintained:

$$\frac{K^+ \text{ (inside)}}{K^+ \text{ (outside)}} = \frac{Cl^- \text{ (outside)}}{Cl^- \text{ (inside)}}.$$

Water osmotically follows the ionic movement of the cell, concentrating the internal K^+, so that even though the cell loses K^+, the intracellular K^+ concentration does not change. The cell loses enough Cl^- to make the ratio $\dfrac{Cl^- \text{ (outside)}}{Cl^- \text{ (inside)}}$, balanced once again and of course equal to $\dfrac{K^+ \text{ (inside)}}{K^+ \text{ (outside)}}$. Consider the consequence for the cell if for some reason it should become permeable to protein anion. What would happen to the charges inside and outside the cell? Fig. 3-1 illustrates these ionic movements, which allow the Gibbs-Donnan relationship to be maintained.

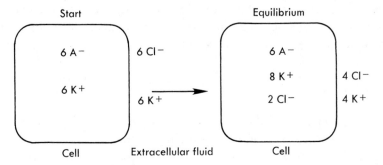

Fig. 3-1. A⁻ ions are nondiffusible cellular anions. At equilibrium, products of diffusible ions are equal ($8 \times 2 = 4 \times 4$), and:

$$\frac{K^+\ (\text{inside})}{K^+\ (\text{outside})} = \frac{Cl^-\ (\text{outside})}{Cl^-\ (\text{inside})} \left(\frac{8}{4} = \frac{4}{2} \right)$$

Since these osmotic particles are inside the cell, it swells.

MEMBRANE POTENTIAL

If recording electrodes are inserted through a cell membrane, and the difference in charge between the inside and the outside is measured, all cells will have some difference in potential, measured in millivolts. Human cells are negatively charged on the inner membrane surface. The magnitude of this potential difference across a membrane depends on the cell type. Excitable cells have greater potential differences in the resting state than nonexcitable cells. This voltage, which is generated across the cell membrane, has several implications. First, it suggests that cells may be able to *conduct* an electrical current. Second, it is a phenomenon that affects the diffusion of molecules, ions, and atoms across the cell membrane, since such diffusion is dependent on the *electro*chemical difference. It also implies that a separation of charge across the membrane must involve a separation of certain charged ions. The distribution of the major body electrolytes and the operation of the Na⁺-K⁺ active transport pump were previously discussed. The pump mechanism keeps the intracellular Na⁺ concentration low and the intracellular K⁺ high, by pumping out any Na⁺ that leaks in and pumping back in any K⁺ that leaks out.

Let us now examine exactly how an electrical difference is generated across a typical excitable cell membrane. This potential is known as the resting membrane potential (RMP). A general abbreviation for the membrane potential is E_m. Since K⁺ concentration is much higher inside the cell, there is a downhill gradient for K⁺ diffusion from inside to outside.

The membrane acts as a barrier to that diffusion, as does the negativity of the membrane. However, some K^+ does of course move to the outside of the cell. The cells and body fluids are subject to physical laws, and therefore an electrical attraction between negatively and positively charged particles is always present. For every positively charged K^+, there is an associated anion, such as Cl^-, SO_4^{-2}, or $H_3PO_4^-$. Inside cells, trapped protein is, at cell pH, anionic; thus it also balances the K^+. At the membrane a charge difference is set up because of the permeability of the membrane to K^+ and its impermeability to cellular anions. As K^+ moves out of the cell, it attracts anions that are not able to diffuse through the membrane. These anions "follow" the K^+ and line up along the inner surface, creating a negatively charged inner membrane. The E_m of any membrane is determined by the most permeable ion that can diffuse through that membrane. For most cells in the resting state that ion is K^+, but a difference is seen in red blood cells, which have a very low permeability to both Na^+ and K^+, and a much greater Cl^- permeability. Thus the red blood cell's membrane potential is due to Cl^- diffusion and is close to the Cl^- *diffusion potential*. This diffusion potential is the potential difference that would develop across the cell membrane if Cl alone were the only ion able to diffuse. Most cells have a largely K^+ diffusion potential. Let us examine what the E_m would be in a cell if K^+ were indeed the only ion that could move across that particular cell's membrane. The E_m would be that potential difference at which the inward and outward movements of K^+ are exactly balanced. In other words, if the membrane potential could be set to the diffusion potential for K^+ (E_{K^+}), then no *net* movement of K^+ could occur. To calculate the E_{K^+}, several things must be known. They are calculated into the *Nernst equation*, the simplified form of which is presented below:

$$E_{K^+} = \frac{RT}{F} \ln \frac{(K^+)\ \text{in}}{(K^+)\ \text{out}}$$

By calculating $\dfrac{RT}{F}$, which is the product of the gas constant and the absolute temperature divided by the faraday (number of coulombs per mole of charge), and converting $\ln$ (the natural logarithm) to the common logarithm, we have a modified Nernst equation, as follows:

$$E_{K^+} = -61.5 \times \log_{10} \frac{(K^+)\ \text{in}}{(K^+)\ \text{out}}$$

It is now necessary to calculate only the intracellular and extracellular concentrations of K^+. This process is fairly simple, and the values can be obtained from Table 2-3. Thus we see that intracellular K^+ is 150 mEq/liter, and extracellular K^+ is 5 mEq/liter. Substituting these values in the Nernst equation:

$$E_K = -61.5 \times \log_{10} \frac{150}{5} = -61.5 \times \log_{10} 30$$

$$E_K = -61.5 \times 1.47 = -90 \text{ mV}$$

Thus the K^+ equilibrium potential is very close to the RMP that is present in most excitable cells, which averages around -90 mV. In any cell it is the *most easily diffusible ion* that determines the E_m, and for most cells this is the K^+ ion.

The effects of altered K^+ diffusion on the E_m are obviously important. Recall that diffusion through a membrane depends on two factors: the electrochemical gradient and the membrane permeability. Thus K^+ diffusion could be altered by changing either the gradient or the membrane permeability, two situations that can be experimentally demonstrated. If the diffusion gradient is decreased, either by increasing the external K^+ concentration or by making the membrane more positive on the outside so that K^+ movement to the outside is electrically impeded, there will be less K^+ diffusion to the outside. Thus, as compared to normal, less negative charge will accumulate along the inner membrane surface, and there will be a drop in potential, or less charge separation, resulting in membrane *depolarization* (less polarization). The opposite occurs when the external K^+ concentration is decreased even less than normal, so that a larger outward diffusion gradient is present. More K^+ diffuses out, more anion lines up along the inner membrane, and the amount of charge separation is greater than normal (i.e., the membrane becomes *hyperpolarized*).

The membrane also becomes hyperpolarized when the membrane permeability to K^+ is increased. Conversely it becomes depolarized if its normal K^+ permeability is decreased. These membrane permeability changes may occur when the lipid composition and fluidity are altered by externally applied agents (e.g., lysolecithin) or in certain disease states (e.g., hemolytic anemias).

The regulation of K^+ movements across cells will be described in much greater detail in the chapter on K^+ imbalances.

ACTION POTENTIAL

The action potential is a self-propagating wave of electrochemical depolarization. When cells become electrically excited and actually transmit an electrochemical message down their length, the basic reason is transitory changes in membrane permeability. Remember that a cell's RMP is determined by the most permeable ion, which is usually K^+. If the Nernst equation is used and it is now assumed that the most permeable ion is Na^+, suddenly the following relationship can be seen:

$$E_m = -61.5 \times \log_{10} \frac{(Na^+)_i}{(Na^+)_o}$$

$$E_m = -61.5 \times \log \frac{10}{145} = 71.4$$

In this case, then, the E_m would rapidly change from -90 mV, the K^+ potential, to a positive sodium potential. This is basically what happens when a cell becomes excited enough to fire an action potential. An action potential is the result of a sudden change in membrane potential, as seen in Fig. 3-2. When a cell "fires," not only does it produce a local action potential, but this electrical change is transmitted along the adjacent membrane and is propagated as far as is anatomically possible. The local potential difference resulting in an action potential is due to a sudden increase in cell membrane permeability to Na^+ at the point of stimulation.

Nerve and muscle cells can be stimulated by many different types of stimuli. Electrical, chemical, and physical stimuli all result in the same phenomenon: an action potential. Of course, the nervous system is designed to efficiently transmit the most appropriate signal. Thus the

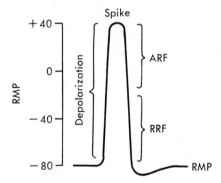

Fig. 3-2. Action potential. Cell depolarizes because of transient increase in Na^+ permeability. Peak of action potential approaches E_{Na^+}, but there is not enough time for the E_{Na^+} of 68 to be reached, and usually, height of spike is $+30$ to $+40$ mV. RMP = Resting membrane potential; ARF = absolute refractory period; RRF = relative refractory period.

optic nerve terminates in an elaborate receptor, the eye, which trans-
duces light energy into action potentials in the fibers of the optic nerve.
However, it is possible to stimulate the optic nerve mechanically. For
example, some blind children may forcefully rub their eyes with their fists,
producing the impression of light flashes called phosphenes. The optic
nerve is stimulated and the visual centers of the brain respond, causing
blind children with intact optic nerves to have the sensation of vision.
Another common example of nonspecific stimulation of sensory receptors
is the annoying sensation produced by aluminum foil or metal on fillings
in the teeth. The touch receptors become electrically stimulated by the
metallic contact, resulting in action potentials in the nerves. The significance of the result of nonspecific stimulation is that excitable cells, when
stimulated by many different types of stimuli of sufficient strength, respond in a uniform way, by action potentials, or not at all.

The quality of the message that the central nervous system receives is
dependent on the frequency of the action potentials transmitted along
the peripheral nerves. It is not, for example, the amplitude of an action
potential that increases when the strength of stimulation of a touch receptor is increased. Rather, it is the *number* of action potentials per unit
of time that increases. The result is that the brain interprets the increased
rate as increased strength of sensory stimuli. For us this interpretation
means the difference between a twinge of discomfort and excruciating
pain.

Another point in the discussion of cellular excitability has now been
reached. Cells that fire action potentials do so only when stimulation
results in a sufficiently great increase in Na^+ permeability. The degree of
depolarization required for the action potential response is different for
each cell type and is known as the *threshold potential*, which must be
reached before firing can occur. A degree of depolarization that is insuf-
ficient to cause firing may nevertheless make the cells transitorily more
excitable, so that if another subthreshold stimulus is applied to the cell
while the cell is in the slightly depolarized state, an action potential could
result. This property is called *summation*, since two subthreshold stimuli
add together to cause the cell to fire an action potential. Referring again
to Fig. 3-2, notice that the peaked waveform of the action potential on the
graph, often called the spike, shows that the membrane potential reaches
a maximum and then begins to drop back toward the RMP. Two phases
of decreased excitability occur as the membrane potential returns to
normal: the absolute refractory period and the relative refractory period.
During these phases of repolarization, either the cell *cannot* be stimulated

by a stimulus of any strength to fire a new action potential (the absolute period), or it can be stimulated only by a greater-than-normal stimulus (the relative period).

The reason that each step of the action potential occurs in relation to biochemical events at the membrane will now be examined. The first stage of the action potential, depolarization to threshold, is due to a sudden, transient increase in Na^+ permeability and a drop in normal K^+ permeability. Na^+ ions are much more highly concentrated in the ECF, and therefore the altered membrane permeability allows Na^+ to rush into the cell by diffusion, causing the cell to become increasingly positive along the inner membrane surface at the point of stimulation. The increase in Na^+ permeability is about 500 times greater than normal. As the threshold potential is reached, a self-stimulating, or autocatalytic, process called the *Hodgkin cycle* occurs. This increase in Na^+ permeability, which results as the membrane becomes depolarized, is depicted as follows:

Membrane depolarization $\rightarrow$ Increase in Na^+ permeability $\rightarrow$
Diffusion of Na^+ $\rightarrow$ Membrane depolarization

This cycle continues as long as the E_m is less than the Na^+ diffusion potential and causes the cell to reach the full height of the spike. At the height of the spike the phenomenon of Na^+ inactivation occurs. It is as if the Na^+ gates, or pores, which had become open, suddenly close. The cell at this time also regains its K^+ permeability and in fact becomes much more permeable to K^+ than normally. Since K^+ diffusion out of the cell then begins to occur very rapidly, the cell membrane becomes increasingly electronegative, and the membrane potential rises back toward its normal value. In fact, an overshoot occurs, and the E_m actually becomes slightly more negative than normal, before returning to the RMP. Excess Na^+ that has leaked into the cell and excess K^+ that has leaked out are now actively transported by the Na^+-K^+ pump. Therefore any tiny concentration changes in these ions that occurred as the result of the action potential are rectified before the next action potential. These electrochemical events that compose the action potential require very little time. In a peripheral nerve ending, an action potential can take as little as 2 msec, whereas in cardiac muscle the longer time of 600 msec is usual.

Compute how many times in a minute a nerve fiber can fire, as compared to a cardiac muscle fiber. You can see that the maximum number of times per minute that a heart muscle fiber can fire is much less. The important implications for cardiac excitability will be discussed in the next section.

How do we know that these biochemical changes occur during the action potential? One piece of evidence for the role of Na^+ comes from an experiment in which excitable cells are bathed in a medium that contains choline ions and that replaces the normal concentration of Na^+. In this case no action potential can be elicited. Also observed experimentally is a dependence of excitability on the external Na^+ concentration. When the concentration is decreased, the amplitude of the action potential is damped, and if the concentration is decreased enough, the cell cannot be stimulated to fire. Another, more indirect piece of evidence is the fact that the peak of the action potential is very similar to the Na^+ potential (E_{Na^+}). The fact that the action potential does not quite reach the E_{Na^+} is probably due (1) to permeability changes that occur, at that voltage, to other ions such as Ca^{++}, and (2) to the limited time available for depolarization.

FACTORS INFLUENCING EXCITABILITY

It has been stated that cellular excitability is determined by the RMP and the threshold and is caused by transient ionic permeability changes. It is possible to experimentally alter both RMP and threshold and thus change cellular excitability. For example, if the RMP is increased (i.e., the cell is made more negative), then more of a millivoltage change is needed to reach threshold. Another way of affecting excitability would be to change the threshold voltage to a more negative or more positive value. In the latter case, a lesser millivoltage change would be needed to fire the cell, whereas in the former case, a greater change would be required.

One way of changing RMP is to alter the K^+ concentration in the fluid bathing the cell. This in vitro situation is analogous to clinical states of hypokalemia and hyperkalemia, since in both cases the ECF K^+ concentration bathing excitable cells is changed. The graph in Fig. 3-3 shows the rise in RMP with decreasing K^+ concentration. As the K^+ drops, a steeper gradient for K^+ diffusion out of the cell and into the bathing medium exists. Since the RMP is the result of K^+ diffusion out of the cell, which causes trapped anions to line up along the inner membrane surface, the RMP becomes more negative as the diffusion of K^+ is enhanced. The cell becomes hyperpolarized and therefore is more difficult to stimulate. Excitability is decreased.

Just the opposite happens, within certain limits, in cells bathed in greater-than-normal K^+ concentration. Diffusion of K^+ out of the cell is limited because the diffusion gradient is less than normal. Therefore less negativity occurs along the inner membrane surface; the cell is partially

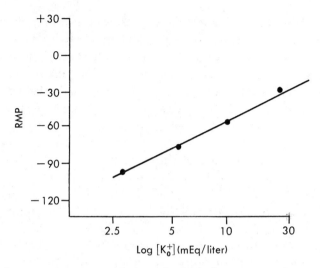

Fig. 3-3. With increasing concentration of external potassium, resting membrane potential (RMP) becomes increasingly positive.

depolarized. The RMP is close to the threshold, and the cell becomes hyperexcitable and is easily fired.

Potassium's major effect is therefore on RMP. Calcium appears to influence threshold, and calcium imbalance (hypocalcemia or hypercalcemia) changes excitability partly through changes in threshold values. Hypercalcemia favors a drop in threshold, whereas hypocalcemia raises threshold. Thus it is more difficult to reach threshold from the normal RMP when hypercalcemia is present and vice versa. When hypercalcemia is combined clinically with hypokalemia, the two electrolyte aberrations combine to create a situation in which the membrane is hyperpolarized and the threshold is more positive. The cellular excitability is therefore profoundly depressed.

In subsequent chapters more complete discussions of electrolyte effects and their clinical manifestations will be presented.

Conduction

Although the transient change in Na^+ permeability explains the development of the action potential, it is necessary to further explore how the action potential results in a traveling wave of depolarization throughout the length of the conducting cell. This wave of electronegativity can actually travel many feet from dendritic endings in peripheral nerves, along the nerve fiber, to the spinal cord or brain. Furthermore the impulse is propagated without decrement. In a way, the nerves resemble conducting wires. Many are wrapped in a lipid insulation, myelin, which is produced by specialized Schwann's cells, which themselves curl around the nerve fiber. The myelin prevents traveling current from leaking out of the depolarized nerve. When the myelin coat is interrupted, current can leak out, a phenomenon that is the physiologic basis for a theory of impulse propagation called *saltatory conduction.* To understand this theory, consider, first, how the initial action potential causes an impulse to begin to be conducted. Recall that at the site of the action potential the Na^+ ions leak in and cause the interior of the membrane to become more positive with respect to the outside. Fig. 3-4 shows that a local area of positivity results in a current flow from right to left and from left to right. The cause is simply the attraction of positive and negative charges; the current moves farther through the membrane as negative is attracted to positive. These localized areas of current are enough to initiate depolarization of the membrane adjacent to the initial site of action potential formation. Once threshold is reached, the Hodgkin cycle is activated and a new action potential forms.

What happens farther down the conducting cell when this action potential occurs? Additional local circuits are set up, leading again to action potentials, and thus the impulse is conducted along the entire length of the neuron. In myelinated nerve, however, the myelin does not allow local circuits to be set up along the bare membrane, although there are bare spots where myelin is absent, called nodes of Ranvier. The current jumps from node to node, very rapidly conducting the impulse down the length of the nerve. Conduction by myelinated nerves is much more rapid than by

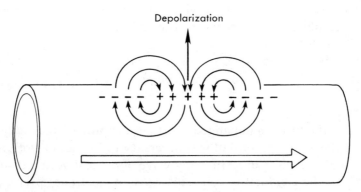

Fig. 3-4. Local circuits arise because of adjacent charge differences along membrane. Result is traveling wave of depolarization.

unmyelinated nerves. The current flows in only one direction because the membrane behind the traveling wave of depolarization is refractory. However, current can flow in either direction from the initial site of depolarization—but it cannot move first forward and then backward. The presence of synapses determines whether the propagated impulse is physiologically significant. It is at the synapse that the directionality of the impulse is manifested. To transmit biologic information, nerve impulses must move across a space, the synapse, and depolarize another cell.

Synaptic transmission

The term *synapse* describes an infinitesimally small (several hundred Angstrom units) space or cleft between two cells, one or both of which are neurons. The presynaptic cell is always a nerve cell, but the postsynaptic cell may be a gland, a muscle, or another nerve. Sensory information from a neuron in a peripheral nerve is transmitted across a synapse in the spinal cord or brain to another neuron, which, in the case of a simple monosynaptic reflex such as the knee jerk, can be a motoneuron. The impulse must in some way affect the postsynaptic cell's membrane to cause depolarization. Looking more closely at the knee jerk, we see that the tendon tap is the stimulus that initially depolarizes neurons, which then conduct the impulse to the spinal cord without decrement. In the spinal cord the neurons, which are presynaptic, synapse with motoneurons that supply the contracting muscles. The impulse moves across the synapse and depolarizes the postsynaptic motoneurons, which then conduct waves of depolarization down to the endings on the muscle units. These motoneurons are now presynaptic to the nerve-muscle synapse. They transmit the impulse across this synapse, and the muscle membrane depolarizes. Through biochemical changes within muscle cells, which will be described later, the muscle contracts.

Fig. 3-5 shows a drawing of a myoneural junction. This incredibly narrow space is the site of amazing events that underlie the process of impulse propagation across the synapse.

For the postsynaptic membrane to become depolarized, it too must become suddenly permeable to Na^+. The wave of depolarization cannot move from the presynaptic cell across the synaptic cleft; chemical messenger substances are released by the nerve impulse from the presynaptic cell. These neurotransmitters are then able to facilitate postsynaptic membrane depolarization by increasing postsynaptic membrane permeability to Na^+. Another aspect of this process is the amplification of the nerve impulse, which is needed before a postsynaptic muscle cell can fire. The

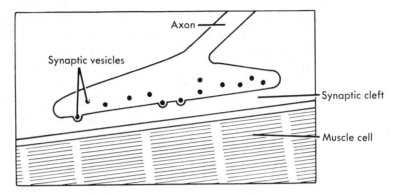

Fig. 3-5. Myoneural synapse is tiny space between nerve endings and muscle cell membrane, across which the neurotransmitter, released from synaptic vesicles, diffuses and depolarizes postsynaptic membrane.

muscle membrane surface area is 1000 times greater than the nerve cell membrane area at the synapse. The way the nerve impulse is amplified and transmitted across the muscle membrane depends on the presence of adequate amounts of chemical transmitter substances, which are stored in vesicles. When the impulse reaches the presynaptic membrane terminals, it causes the vesicles to be extruded into the synaptic cleft and ruptured open to release the neurotransmitter. This process appears to be linked to an increased Ca^{++} permeability, which allows the vesicles to be extruded by exocytosis. Mg^{++} inhibits this process. The postsynaptic membrane has many specific receptor sites for the neurotransmitter. Once the chemical substance binds with and saturates these receptors, a dramatic increase in Na^+ permeability ensues. The mechanism by which the increase in Na^+ permeability occurs is not known. Much research has been aimed at identifying and isolating membrane receptor sites in an attempt to understand the basic physiology of nerve-muscle transmission and also to find new treatments for diseases such as myasthenia gravis and muscular dystrophy.

Drug effects

Researchers have learned a great deal about the synapse through the use of various drugs affecting transmission. For example, curare, a chemical first used by Indians in South America, who placed the drug on tips of spears to paralyze their enemies, is now used medically. Curare appears to act by binding to postsynaptic receptor sites for a common neurotransmitter, acetylcholine. By thus saturating the postsynaptic membrane, curare blocks the depolarizing action of acetylcholine. Thus the muscle cell cannot depolarize, and no contractions are possible. Succinylcholine is another drug that acts in the same way. These drugs are used to promote muscle relaxation during surgery, so that lesser amounts of general anesthetic agents are then required.

Other drugs known to alter synaptic transmission are classified as *cholinesterase inhibitors*. Cholinesterase is an enzyme that degrades acetylcholine almost as soon as it is released into the synaptic cleft; thus the neurotransmitter's action is very brief. Drugs that inhibit cholinesterase therefore allow the action of acetylcholine to be prolonged. Examples of drugs with this action are eserine (physostigmine) and neostigmine (Prostigmin).

Neurotransmitters

The ability of the postsynaptic cell to fire an action potential depends on an adequate amount of neurotransmitter molecules. Before postsynaptic cells can repolarize and not be refractory when another impulse arrives at the synapse, the neurotransmitters must be removed. Acetylcholine is enzymatically destroyed within the synaptic cleft, as was previously mentioned, and very small amounts are again taken into the presynaptic cell. This method is more important in neurotransmitter removal for certain other transmitter subtances, such as norepinephrine, the major transmitter substance of the sympathetic nervous system. Within the brain, many other neurotransmitters, some excitatory and others inhibitory, have been identified. The list includes gamma-aminobutyric acid (GABA), glycine, dopamine, glutamic acid, serotonin, and histamine, and other neurotransmitters are being discovered constantly. Researchers have even learned recently that gut hormones (e.g., secretin, gastrin) may have a neurotransmitter role in the brain, which apparently produces these substances endogenously.

Exciting research has shown how certain neurotransmitters are responsible for feelings of elation and well-being, whereas others dictate depression and gloominess. It is now known that many drugs that alter mood act at the synaptic level to influence neurotransmitter activity.

MECHANISM OF MUSCLE CONTRACTION

The anatomic arrangement of nerve and muscle is known as the motor unit. It is composed of a nerve cell and all the muscle cells that it innervates. The implication is that for skeletal muscle the ratio of nerve fiber to muscle cell is not 1:1. More commonly, in a large leg muscle, for

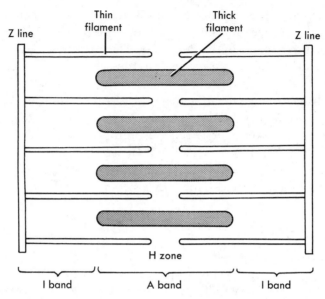

Fig. 3-6. Muscle filaments are arranged in units known as sarcomeres—distance between two Z lines.

example, there may be 100 muscle cells to a single motor nerve cell. The arrival of a nerve impulse at a postsynaptic muscle cell results in a series of biochemical events that culminate in the contraction of the muscle cell. The electrophysiology of the three muscle types differs significantly. However, the basic biochemistry of all types of muscular contraction appears to be very similar and involves the sliding of molecular filaments of actin and myosin. The sliding filament theory of muscular contraction will be described as it applies to skeletal muscle, since the process has been best characterized in this context. Fig. 3-6 is a drawing of a muscle fiber with intense striations. These striations are due to the bending of polarized light by the structural arrangement of molecules within the muscle cell. The names of each dark and light band are indicated. The physiologic unit of muscle contraction is the distance between two Z lines and is known as the *sarcomere*. Muscle contraction is the result of a shortening of sarcomeres of individual muscle fibers, a phenomenon producing the sliding of filaments that make up the sarcomere. The filaments are composed of two major muscle proteins, actin and myosin. Thin filaments are composed of actin, and myosin molecules make up the thick filaments. Fig. 3-6 shows how thick and thin filaments are arranged within a sarcomere. Actin filaments are joined to the Z lines. During muscular contraction the Z lines move together, approaching the ends of the A band, and the I band disappears. This shortening is the result of a sliding of actin filaments along myosin filaments, and in extreme contraction the actin filaments actually overlap each other at the center of the A band.

The molecular mechanism of the filament sliding is important to understand because these processes may be altered in certain fluid and electrolyte abnormalities. The normal process involves energy expenditure and a supply of Ca^{++}.

The system of filament sliding is powered by the hydrolysis of adenosine triphosphate (ATP) to adenosine diphosphate (ADP) and inorganic phosphate. Of course, this ATP is obtained through glucose metabolism by the muscle cells. Muscle fibers shorten during contraction, an effect produced by the sliding of thick and thin filaments. Fibers lengthen during relaxation as the filaments slide back to their resting positions in preparation for the next contraction. It is the release of Ca^{++} into the interior of the cell that initiates filament sliding. Depolarization of the muscle cell membrane, through excitation-contraction coupling, causes sequestered Ca^{++} to suddenly become available to the sliding filament mechanism. Almost as soon as the Ca^{++} is released from the specialized intracellular tubular system that contains it, it is taken up again, so that its action is extremely short lived. Therefore contraction of a muscle fiber is very brief and is known as a twitch.

Ca^{++} functions in the hydrolysis of ATP, which is necessary to provide energy for thin filaments to slide over thick filaments. Myosin makes up thick filaments, and the heads of these molecules form connections, known as cross-bridges, between thick and thin filaments. For sliding to occur, the cross-bridges must move. Cross-bridges are normally coated by molecules of an inhibitory protein, tropomyosin. Troponin, an inhibitor attached to actin, forms a complex with tropomyosin. This complex prevents the myosin cross-bridges from moving. However, when the muscle cell membrane becomes depolarized, and Ca^{++} is released into the interior of the cell, the inhibiting proteins are removed from the heads of the myosin molecules. It is believed that Ca^{++} binds with troponin, causing movement of the tropomyosin molecules away from the myosin. This action, then, exposes the myosin cross-bridges. Myosin not only is a structural muscle protein but is also able to act as an enzyme. When the myosin heads are exposed, myosin acts enzymatically as an adenosinetriphosphatase (ATPase), an enzyme that catalyzes ATP hydrolysis. The energy so released results in movement of the cross-bridges in a ratchetlike action by which actin filaments slide over myosin filaments. As long as Ca^{++} is present, contraction of muscle fibers continues.

Ca^{++} release and uptake are accomplished by internal membrane tubular systems located inside muscle cells. These systems are the T system and the sarcoplasmic reticulum (SR). The T system conducts the action potential into the interior of the cell and stimulates the release of Ca^{++} from the SR. After it is released, active transport immediately operates to pump Ca^{++} back into the SR, allowing muscle relaxation to occur.

This complex, elegant system is the basis for muscular contraction in skeletal, smooth, and cardiac muscle. Differences between the three muscle types do exist, particularly with regard to excitability characteristics.

Smooth and cardiac muscle properties

Whereas skeletal muscle requires external stimulation to contract, smooth and cardiac muscles have the property of *automaticity*. These muscles contract rhythmically and independently of outside stimuli. Although outside nervous control of smooth and cardiac muscle is present, it acts mainly as a regulator of the muscular contractions. Thus the vagus nerve and sympathetic fibers both have effects on cardiac rhythm and contraction strength, but the heart is well able to beat in the absence of innervation, a fact well supported by the numerous heart transplant patients, whose hearts have absolutely no direct nervous system control! Another unique property of both smooth and cardiac muscle is conductivity. These muscle fibers are able to transmit waves of depolarization from one muscle cell to the other without any known intermediary chemical transmitters. Thus the electrical message moves rapidly through groups of smooth muscle fibers, with sequential excitation followed by contraction. Peristalsis is an excellent example of this type of conductivity. Most smooth muscle excitation is initiated by specialized muscle cells known as pacemaker cells. The same is true for cardiac contraction. The pacemaker cell has an innate biologic rhythm of electrical depolarization. This focus of depolarization is the initiating site of the wave of depolarization that results in contraction. Pacemakers are known to exist within the cardiovascular system and the gastrointestinal, urinary, and reproductive tracts, all of which contain smooth or cardiac muscle. The rate of discharge from pacemaker cells may be profoundly influenced by the neural and chemical milieu, as best examplified by the cardiac pacemaker regulation. The sinoatrial (SA) node, which is located in the right atrium of the heart, functions normally as the pacemaker for the heartbeat, which is within the range of 60 to 100 beats/min for both women and men. When an individual is excited, nervous, or stressed, the heart rate increases because of the effect of sympathetic nervous system arousal. Sympathetic fibers transmit impulses to the SA node, increasing the slope of the pacemaker potential so that impulse firing becomes more frequent, causing the heart rate to speed up to rates occasionally in excess of 200 beats/min. Another example of nervous control over automaticity is reflected in biofeedback experiments. Yogis and some trained individuals are able to decrease their resting heart rate remarkably through conscious effort. These persons have "learned" to increase the rate of firing of the vagus nerve, which normally slows the heart, or perhaps to suppress the sympathetic nervous system. Heart rate can be decreased to 30 beats/min in some cases.

Many of the common fluid and electrolyte imbalances can have profound effects on smooth and cardiac muscle automaticity and conductivity. The patient with hypokalemia, for example, often has symptoms of decreased gastrointestinal motility. Since potassium is the major ion responsible for the RMP, when external K^+ is decreased, a larger diffusion gradient from the inside to the outside of the cell occurs. More K^+ tends to leave the cell, and therefore more anion lines up on the inner membrane surface, hyperpolarizing the smooth muscle cells of the gut. This hyperpolarization of course makes it more difficult to stimulate these cells to contract; thus peristaltic waves do not pass as readily through the length of the gut. Patients with severe hypokalemia may develop intestinal obstruction.

This book describes many other examples of fluid and electrolyte effects on cellular physiology and the resultant disruptions of normal organ function.

4

Renal physiology and pathophysiology

The kidneys are the major water excretory organs. Their structure is complex and highly differentiated, the anatomy providing an example of how well structure is correlated with function. Located in the retroperitoneal area of the flank, the kidneys are protected from abdominal insult by the bony protection of the rib cage. It is difficult to palpate the kidneys through the abdomen even by deep palpation, but occasionally the right kidney may be felt during deep inspiration by the patient.

GROSS ANATOMY

The gross anatomy of the right kidney is diagramed in Fig. 4-1. The renal cortex comprises the outer layers of cells; the medulla is the more inward layer. Notice that the urinary calices in the medulla are formed from the merging of the collecting ducts of the separate nephrons. The *nephron* is the anatomic and physiologic unit of the kidney and consists of a blood filter (the glomerulus) and a tubular system that collects the blood filtrate, processes it, and produces urine. The collecting ducts empty into the calices, which then drain into a larger tube, called the *ureter*, leading from the kidney to the bladder. The kidneys themselves are small, weighing about 140 gm in the adult. They are bean shaped, highly vascular, and protected by a connnective tissue capsule. The total mass of renal tissue necessary for adequate renal function is much less than that normally present. Normal renal physiology can be maintained even when only 20% of the kidney tissue is present. When kidney disease or destruction occurs, the remaining kidney tissue hypertrophies and becomes more efficient. This fact makes renal transplant a possibility, since no deficit appears to occur in a person with only one kidney.

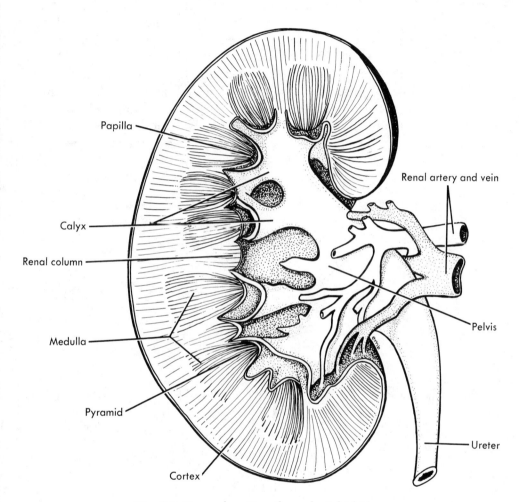

Fig. 4-1. Coronal section through right kidney.

MICROSCOPIC ANATOMY

The nephron consists of a unique arrangement of epithelial cells in close association with the microvasculature of the kidney. Fig. 4-2 presents the micropscopic anatomy of a model nephron. The glomerulus is a tuft of capillaries across which the filtering of the blood occurs. This filtrate, which is very similar to protein-free plasma, enters into a cuplike collecting structure known as Bowman's capsule. The filtrate then drains into a tubule, known as the *proximal convoluted tubule* (PCT), leading from Bowman's capsule. The plasma filtrate undergoes chemical change in the PCT by the processes of reabsorption and secretion. Some substances move out of the filtrate through the epithelial lining cells of the PCT and into the renal interstitium. The latter is in diffusion equilibrium with the blood in the peritubular capillaries; thus substances eventually

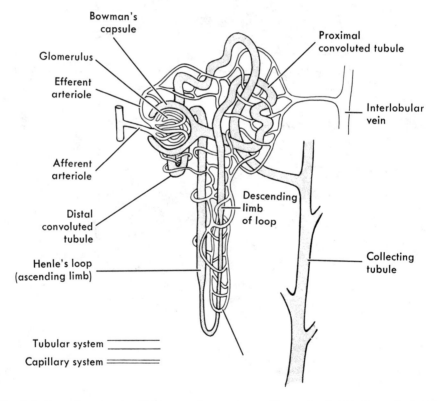

Fig. 4-2. Functional unit of kidney—the nephron. (From Groër, M. E., and Shekleton, M. E.: Basic pathophysiology: a conceptual approach, St. Louis, 1979, The C. V. Mosby Co.)

move into the bloodstream as the result of this reabsorption process. Other substances are secreted into the filtrate from the blood, through the renal tubular epithelium. This epithelial lining is composed of a thin single layer of cells, and diffusion across this barrier readily occurs for most substances. These cells are the only barrier separating the tubular filtrate from the interstitium. The endothelial lining of the peritubular capillaries represents a second barrier for movement into and out of the capillary blood, but it also is highly permeable and does not inhibit diffusion to any great degree.

After the PCT the remainder of the nephron consists of the *loop of Henle*, which is formed by a descending limb and an ascending limb of Henle. The loops of Henle are either fairly short or, in 20% of nephrons, very long, dipping down into the medulla. The significance of this difference in length will be discussed later. As the filtrate moves through the loop of Henle, reabsorption and secretion continue to change the filtrate into actual urine. The ascending limb terminates in the *distal convoluted tubule* (DCT), which empties into the collecting duct. The completion of the process of urine formation takes place in the collecting ducts, and urine moves into the ureters. The urine undergoes no other major change as it drains into the bladder through the ureters, unless some pathologic condition exists.

RENAL BLOOD FLOW

Before considering in detail the processes of filtration, reabsorption, and secretion, we must closely examine the relationship of renal blood flow (RBF) to renal physiology. The major artery supplying blood to the kidney is the renal artery, which branches from the aorta. The renal artery then subdivides into the *arcuate* arteries, which further branch into *interlobular* arteries. These then subdivide into the *afferent* arterioles that supply each nephron. The afferent arterioles lead into a tuft of capillaries, called the *glomerulus*, within Bowman's capsule. The glomerulus eventually forms an *efferent* arteriole that drains the blood from the glomerulus. The kidney is unusual in that a double capillary system is present: the efferent arteriole breaks into a system of peritubular capillaries, which eventually drain the blood into the interlobular veins. The venous system drains the blood from the kidney and empties into the inferior vena cava.

The RBF is measured in several different ways, such as by the clearance of dyes and chemicals accomplished by the kidney in one pass of the blood through that organ. Various techniques have demonstrated that

RBF is about 1200 ml/min (one fifth of the cardiac output) in man. All of this blood passes through the glomerular capillaries in the manner just described. The RBF is determined by several factors, including the hydrostatic pressure of the blood as it is ejected into the aorta during ventricular systole. Another major variable affecting RBF is the resistance to blood flow that is offered by the renal blood vessels, which are controlled both by the sympathetic nervous system and through intrinsic autoregulation. Under most phsyiologic conditions the resistance of the blood vessels does not change markedly, since the RBF is amazingly constant. The sympathetic nervous system supplies mainly the afferent arteriole, and activation of these nerves results in vasoconstriction. In addition, parasympathetic nerves supplying the efferent arteriole release acetylcholine and are vasodilative in action.

The kidney is able to maintain RBF by autoregulation even when the nerves to the kidney are severed. In this process renal perfusion is maintained even when systemic blood pressure is decreased or elevated. Local mechanisms appear to be responsible for the effect. Autoregulation is in some way related to renal metabolism. Metabolic waste products, prostaglandins, renin-angiotensin, and a local response to vessel stretch have each been suggested, but no one mechanism has been definitely shown to control autoregulation. There is no question that the phenomenon occurs, but its local control is still a subject of research.

GLOMERULAR FILTRATION RATE

In general the ability of the kidney to maintain its RBF is constant even when blood pressure changes occur. However, RBF is affected by conditions that result in intense sympathetic nervous system activity, such as might occur in shock, life-threatening hypoxia, severe pain, or certain behavioral states such as anger or fright. In these cases RBF does decrease. The net effect of decreased RBF is on the *glomerular filtration rate* (GFR), which is the rate of filtration of plasma across the glomerulus into Bowman's capsule. Human studies have shown that the normal male GFR is 125 ml/min/1.73 sq m, and the female value is 10% less. This rate can be maintained by functional nephrons when as much as 50% of the kidney is diseased. To compensate, the functional nephrons hypertrophy and increase filtration across the glomeruli. GFR begins to drop when two thirds of the normal number of nephrons is absent or diseased, and the kidneys at this point become less able to perform their excretory function. A rise in the blood urea nitrogen (BUN) and in creatinine reflects

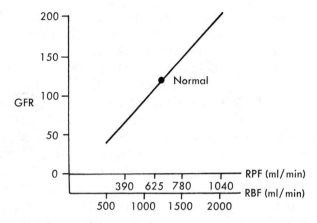

Fig. 4-3. GFR varies directly with RBF, both being increased by dilation of afferent arteriole. Slightly less than half of RBF is plasma flow (approximately 625 ml/min), and proportion of GFR to renal plasma flow (RPF) is known as filtration fraction.

the degree of this inadequacy. These relationships will be explored in a later section dealing with acute renal failure.

Fig. 4-3 shows the relationship of GFR to RBF. It is apparent that the RBF in fact controls GFR to a large degree. Filtration across the glomerular endothelium is not strikingly different from that occurring across capillaries elsewhere in the body. Net filtration is dependent on the Starling capillary forces described in Chapter 2. The major filtering force is due to the hydrostatic pressure of the blood, a pressure controlled by gravity forces. Thus the actual weight and amount of the blood and the dynamic force of that blood as it is ejected from the left ventricle into the arterial tree will be the ultimate factors in determining the effective filtration pressure across the glomerulus. There is normally little tissue pressure resistance to glomerular filtration, and the major opposing force for glomerular filtration is therefore colloid osmotic pressure of the glomerular capillary blood. The reason is that plasma proteins are trapped within the glomerulus, being too large to diffuse out of this membrane into Bowman's capsule. The glomerular filtering membrane is, however, much more permeable than other capillary membranes.

The pressure of the blood in the afferent arteriole is nearly twice that of the systemic arterioles because less resistance is offered by these short, wide vessels. This pressure is a force that favors filtration. Another factor in filtration is the high resistance offered by the efferent arterioles, which are narrow and long. It is obvious that changes in the radii of these vessels will affect GFR. For example, when the afferent arterioles are constricted by increased sympathetic nervous system activity or autoregulation, there is an increased resistance to blood flow. The pressure will therefore drop in the glomeruli, causing a decrease in the filtering-out force and a corresponding drop in GFR. Conversely, if the afferent arteriole dilates, both the blood hydrostatic pressure in the glomerulus and the GFR increase. Constriction of the efferent arteriole causes an increased resistance to blood flow out of the glomerulus. The blood pressure increases within the glomerulus because of this resistance, and the result is an increased GFR. Obviously, when the efferent arteriole vasodilates, the glomerular pressure dissipates and less filtration takes place. Note, however, that alterations in the GFR caused by vascular changes in the efferent arteriole will have opposite effects on the RBF. Constriction of the efferent arteriole, for example, increases GFR, but as a result of the resistance to blood flow offered by these vessels, an eventual drop in RBF occurs.

Since the first step in the formation of urine is filtration, it is important to understand the nature of the forces that govern it. The net filtration out of the glomerular capillaries is determined by the blood hydrostatic pressure and the tissue colloid osmotic pressure. This value is small in Bowman's capsule, since very little protein filters into the fluid here. However, there is an effect opposing filtration that is due to the fluid hydrostatic pressure in Bowman's capsule. A probable value for the hydrostatic pressure in Bowman's capsule is about 10 mm Hg. The blood pressure in the afferent arteriole is estimated by some to be 45 mm Hg, and the osmotic pressure of the blood is 20 mm Hg. Thus the effective filtering force at the afferent end of the arteriole is 45 − (10 + 20), or 15 mm Hg. At the efferent end of the glomerulus, the pressures remain the same except for a rise in the plasma colloid osmotic pressure to 35 mm Hg. The reason is that fluid lost into Bowman's capsule results in a concentration of the blood in the glomerulus, which results in a rise in the osmotic pressure and also in the *hematocrit* (percentage of red blood cells per deciliter of whole blood). Thus the greatest amount of filtration through the glomerular membrane occurs at the afferent end.

Interference with GFR

The GFR, as we have stated previously, depends on the maintenance of adequate RBF, since it is by the rate of blood flow that the hydrostatic pressure of the blood in the glomerulus is maintained. A drop in RBF results in the delivery of less blood into the afferent arteriole, and therefore GFR drops. When the arterial pressure drops below 90 mm Hg, the GFR is also affected, since autoregulation begins to fail at this level of systemic pressure. Other factors that may influence the Starling forces in the glomerular capillary dynamics include obstructive uropathy, which causes an increase in pressure throughout the system of nephrons and gives rise to increased pressure within the tubules and Bowman's capsule. A kidney stone that becomes lodged in the ureter and that does not permit the passage of urine from that kidney results in a back pressure that opposes GFR, and eventually the kidney may no longer filter at all (renal shutdown).

There are many other situations that may interfere with GFR. Kidney disease and damage to the capillaries of the glomerulus, such as occur in glomerulonephritis, will decrease GFR. Pathophysiologic processes (e.g., liver disease, starvation) that result in hypoalbuminemia can increase GFR, since there will be less osmotic force holding plasma water in the glomerular blood. Dehydration, on the other hand, often results in concentration of the components of the plasma, and the colloid osmotic pressure will therefore increase, which in turn inhibits water movement out of the glomerular blood into Bowman's capsule. The blood pressure also may drop in severe dehydration. Other variables that may result in alterations in the GFR are diseases that affect the permeability of the glomerular filtering membrane. An example is *nephrosis*, a condition in which the glomerular membrane becomes abnormally permeable to proteins, with the effects of dissipating the blood colloid osmotic pressure and increasing GFR. An additional effect of this pathologic interference is that a state of hypoalbuminemia develops, and edema in other body tissues results.

Clearance studies

Although the rate of GFR is an important value clinically, the effectiveness of GFR is measured by clearance studies. Experimental studies have utilized *inulin* clearance as the baseline. Inulin is a sugarlike molecule filtered at the glomerulus. Its filtration is very efficient, and its rate of clearance equals the GFR. The following formula is used to measure the clearance of any substance:

$$C = \frac{U \times V}{P} \qquad\qquad 1$$

Clearance is equal to the urinary concentration of a given substance multiplied by the urine volume excreted per minute and divided by the plasma concentration of that substance. In the case of inulin, the amount filtered at the glomerulus is a reflection of the GFR, since the molecule is not processed in any way as it moves through renal tubules. The normal urine output in the adult is 1 ml/min. Therefore in equation 1:

$$C_{inulin} = \frac{U_{inulin} \times 1 \text{ ml/min}}{P_{inulin}} \qquad \qquad 2$$

When the real values for plasma inulin concentration and urine inulin concentration are applied, it is seen that 1.25 mg/min of inulin is excreted in the urine, and if the plasma concentration is 0.01 mg/ml, the clearance value of 125 ml/min is obtained. This value is the rate of inulin clearance and also reflects the GFR. It essentially means that 125 ml of plasma has been cleared of 1.25 mg of inulin and that this clearance took place over a time period of 1 minute. Obviously the clearance of a substance will reflect the GFR only if the amount filtered is not changed during its transit through the tubules, collecting ducts, ureters, and bladder.

Clinically, another clearance value, the *creatinine clearance*, is usually determined to measure GFR. Creatinine is produced in the body as a waste product of muscle metabolism. It is filtered efficiently at the glomerulus, and its clearance value closely reflects the GFR. Thus creatinine clearance is the most common measurement of kidney function in that it measures the overall effectiveness of all glomeruli in the filtering process. A reduced value is seen in many kidney diseases in which glomerular function is reduced. A point should be made about the manner of determination of the creatinine clearance. The nurse must carefully weigh the patient to determine the likely normal value for an individual of that size. The urine is collected over a 24-hour period. It is important to determine this time span accurately, since the creatinine clearance will be underestimated if the period of collection is less than 24 hours.

TUBULAR REABSORPTION

Once the plasma filtrate moves into the tubules of the nephron, great changes in its composition occur as the result of reabsorption and secretion. Reabsorption of filtered substances occurs along the length of the nephron, but the greatest amount occurs in the PCT. The substances that are reabsorbed include Na^+, K^+, Ca^{++}, Mg^{++}, NH_4^+, Cl^-, HCO_3^-, phosphate, sulfate, glucose, amino acids, urea, ascorbic acid, and other molecules to varying degrees. Reabsorption is largely dictated by the body needs and thus is carefully regulated. Part of this regulation is a function of concentration effects alone, but reabsorption is also controlled by various hormones such as parathyroid hormone and aldosterone.

General characteristics

The reabsorption process involves the movement of molecules and ions through the luminal membrane of the cells lining the tubule. The characteristics of this membrane are the subject of much investigation. The cells of the PCT, for example, are now known to have a distinctive luminal surface, which is covered with microvilli. These cellular projections play a role in "catching" transportable molecules in the filtrate as it moves through the PCT and in increasing surface area. Since some pinocytosis also takes place in the PCT, any large molecules that have escaped through the glomerular membrane into the filtrate can be removed almost immediately and are therefore not excreted in the urine. It is important to delineate the passive permeability properties of the luminal membrane of the PCT. Approximately 65% to 80% of the reabsorption of Na^+ occurs in the PCT and is not dependent on hormonal or other regulation but rather appears to be a function of (1) the permeability of the PCT membrane for Na^+ and (2) the diffusion gradient that exists between the Na^+ concentration of the tubular filtrate and that of the tubular cells. Recall that there is normally a low concentration of Na^+ inside cells and that higher amounts occur in the extracellular fluid (ECF). Tubular filtrate is very similar to plasma with respect to the concentrations of the various small solutes normally present in plasma. Therefore a gradient for diffusion into the luminal cells occurs. Fig. 4-4 diagrams the steps involved in the transport of Na^+. Renal cells behave like other cells when excess Na^+ diffuses into them. Active Na^+ transport pumps the excess Na^+ out of the cell and into the ECF. The same process occurs in the PCT, except that there is a polarity of structure and function of these cells. In appearance and action the luminal membrane is entirely different from the membrane facing the interstitial (peritubular) fluid. Since Na^+-K^+-ATPase is present in high concentrations in the peritubular membrane, the net outward pumping occurs only across this membrane of the tubular cells. Na^+ diffuses in one side of the cell and is pumped out the other side of the cell. The luminal and peritubular membranes differ also in the distribution of membrane charges. In the PCT peritubular membrane, there is an E_m of 0 mV, and the E_m is basically determined by the diffusion of K^+ and Cl^-. There is a −20 mV difference across the luminal membrane of the PCT, and the inside is negative with respect to the outside. Here the E_m is deter-

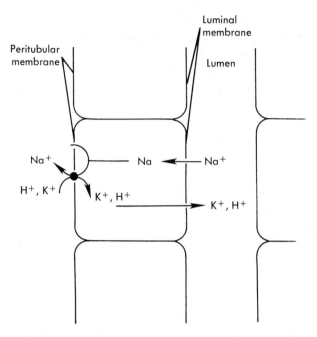

Fig. 4-4. Na^+ diffuses from filtrate through luminal membrane and into cell. It is pumped out through peritubular membrane and is subsequently diffused into renal capillary blood and reabsorbed into systemic circulation. K^+ and H^+ move in opposite direction, their movement's being linked to Na^+ reabsorption.

mined primarily by the diffusion of Na^+. This electrochemical polarity is also maintained in the DCT, but the magnitude of the luminal potential increases to -50 mV. Remember that diffusion is dependent on the electrochemical gradient, and therefore the movement of positively charged substances is facilitated by the negativity of the membrane. Na^+ diffusion is a major phenomenon of the PCT because of its concentration gradient and the electrochemical potential of the luminal membrane.

Tubular maximum

Another important substance that is reabsorbed in the PCT is glucose. Normally there is no glucose present in the urine, indicating that all of the glucose present in the tubular filtrate (basically that of plasma, or 80 to 120 mg/dl) is reabsorbed. The process of glucose reabsorption is not completely understood, but several concepts have resulted from its study. The rate of reabsorption of a substance, called the *tubular maximum* (T_m) is one of the concepts to be discussed. Glucose reabsorption is through an active transport, energy-requiring mechanism, or pump, located at the luminal surface of the cells of the PCT. This active transport mechanism efficiently moves all of the glucose present in the tubular filtrate at normal physiologic concentrations of plasma (and thus filtrate) glucose. However, when glucose concentration rises to high values, the amount of glucose presented to the transporting system exceeds the transport ability of that system. The carrier system is saturated with glucose molecules and is working at its maximum rate and efficiency. The maximum amount of glucose that can be transported per minute is referred to as the T_m for glucose. The usual value is *340 mg/min* (range of 300 to 375 mg/min). This saturation occurs when the plasma glucose exceeds 300 mg/dl. The most classic demonstration of the T_m is in the hyperglycemic diabetic. One criterion for diagnosing diabetes is the presence of glucose in the urine (glycosuria). Assuming normal kidney function, glycosuria indicates that the glucose transport system is saturated, a phenomenon that occurs only when there is a very high concentration of glucose in the plasma and filtrate. There is evidence that glucose reabsorption is related to Na^+ reabsorption, and the T_m for glucose may be changed by alterations in Na^+ and water uptake.

Other substances that are reabsorbed appear to have T_m, or saturation capacity, indicating that there is a maximum rate of transport for different substances and that it is genetically determined and species-specific. Substances that are reabsorbed through the luminal membrane by carrier mechanisms, usually active transport systems, move out of the tubular cells by diffusion, and again the movement is into the peritubular fluid, not back into the tubular filtrate. This direction of movement also reflects the polarity of the lining tubular cells and the great differences between the luminal membranes and the peritubular membranes. The T_m has been identified for ascorbic acid (vitamin C), amino acids, phosphate, sulfate, and several other natural and artificial injected substances.

Regulation of reabsorption

The substances reabsorbed along the length of the nephron are regulated to differing degrees. Obviously, the needs of the body dictate the extent of reabsorption. Another important variable with regard to reabsorption is the hydration state of the body. When the body is dehydrated, reabsorption of water, which partly takes place through increased sodium reabsorption, will increase. The increase in sodium reabsorption causes an osmosis of water with the sodium, and thus less urine is excreted. Regulation of reabsorption of some crucial substances, the concentrations of which influence physiologic function in many important ways, will be discussed below.

Sodium-potassium reabsorption. A general rule with regard to sodium and potassium is that there is net reabsorption of Na^+, but K^+ is usually excreted. The balance of Na^+ within the body fluids is important, but there is a fairly wide range of tolerance before physiologic effects occur. However, K^+ concentration requires much more careful "fine tuning," since there are drastic effects on many functions when small excesses or deficits develop. Therefore any degree of renal failure usually has associated with it an increase in concentration of K^+, which leads to many signs and symptoms (Chapter 8). Renal failure will be discussed later in this chapter.

Sodium reabsorption in the PCT has already been described as the result of purely passive electrochemical gradients. The remainder of the sodium reabsorption occurs in the DCT, loop of Henle, and collecting ducts. Two thirds of the net Na^+ reabsorption is complete when the filtrate leaves the PCT. An important observation about Na^+ reabsorption in the PCT is that an equivalent number of negative anions are reabsorbed along with the Na^+, the major type being bicarbonate anions. The Na^+ movement in the loop of Henle will be described later in the section on countercurrent exchange. The DCT has a limited capacity to transport Na^+, and Na^+ reabsorption is associated here either with anion reabsorption or with net secretion of positive cations to balance the positive charge removed from the filtrate for every Na^+ reabsorbed. The two cations secreted into the filtrate when Na^+ is reabsorbed are K^+ and H^+.

There are probably several transport pathways for Na^+ in the DCT and collecting ducts. There is evidence for the existence of two pumps. Pump 1 is sensitive to the chemical *ethacrynic acid*, which is the active component of a commonly prescribed diuretic, furosemide (Lasix). This pump actively transports Na^+ out of the peritubular membrane and into the interstitial space. It is not a linked pump, and thus its effect is not only to pump out Na^+ but also to pump out positive charges from the cell. Thus it is known as an electrogenic pump, since it creates a negatively charged cell membrane. Pump 2 is a typical Na^+-K^+–linked pump that actively transports Na^+ out of the peritubular membrane and actively transports, in a coupled fashion, K^+ into the cell. K^+ (or H^+) then diffuses into the luminal fluid and may be excreted into the urine. There is a degree of competition between H^+ and K^+ for this pump, so that when excesses of either substance develop, that substance is more likely to be transported from the plasma into the urine as Na^+ is being reabsorbed. This accounts for the hyperkalemia that may develop in acidotic individuals, since the excess H^+ is transported into the urine while the K^+ remains behind in the plasma. Pump 2 is sensitive to the drug *ouabain*, which is a cardiac glycoside with actions similar to those of digitalis. It can be seen that inhibition of either of these pumps will result in less Na^+ reabsorption. The excess Na^+ left in the tubular filtrate will then exert an osmotic effect, causing less water to be reabsorbed through the luminal cells. The net urine output will increase, and the effect is diuretic. Drugs that inhibit these pumps are commonly prescribed for individuals with edematous conditions resulting, for example, from congestive heart failure or kidney disease.

Sodium reabsorption is influenced by several factors. The rate of reabsorption, for example, increases when the GFR increases, although the mechanism for this regulation is not known. Na^+ reabsorption is also decreased when the blood hydrostatic pressure is increased or the plasma proteins are decreased. This decrease of Na^+ may be caused by an opposition to the entry of Na^+ and water into the peritubular capillaries. In fact, there is evidence that a *back leak* of Na^+ and water through spaces between the luminal cells may occur when the capillary blood hydrostatic pressure increases or when blood colloid osmotic pressure decreases. The net effect in either of these conditions would be a diuresis of water along with sodium.

An additional regulation of Na^+ reabsorption is through the hormone *aldosterone*, as well as other adrenocortical steroid hormones to a lesser degree. Aldosterone is released from the cortex of the adrenal gland in response to a complex signaling system, diagramed in Fig. 4-5. The release of aldosterone is ultimately determined by the kidney, which releases the substance *renin*. There are several stimuli to renin release. The cells that release this substance are in the juxtaglomerular apparatus (JGA). The JGA is formed by a thickening of the afferent arteriole caused by hypertrophy of the cells. Adjacent to the JGA, and lying between the afferent and efferent arterioles (Fig. 4-6), is the *macula densa*, a thickening of the wall of the distal tubule as it comes in contact with the JGA and Bowman's capsule. The cells of the JGA are in contact with the macula densa, and evidence for diffusion out of the macula densa and into the afferent arteriole has been presented. The JGA and macula densa together compose the *juxtaglomerular complex*. It has been speculated that Na^+ alterations in the cells of the macula densa, caused by changes in distal tubular fluid, result in stimulation or inhibition of the release of renin from the JGA. Renin can be released either into the blood of the afferent arteriole or into the renal interstitial space, from which it will then diffuse

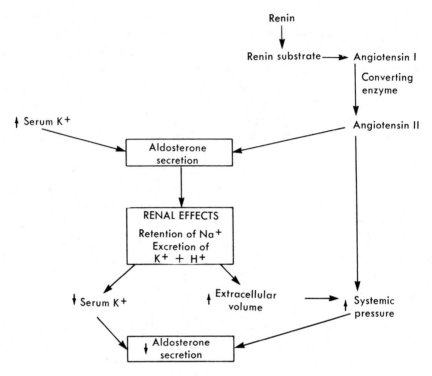

Fig. 4-5. Feedback regulation of aldosterone via two distinct mechanisms. (From Groër, M. E., and Shekleton, M. E.: Basic pathophysiology: a conceptual approach, St. Louis, 1979, The C. V. Mosby Co.)

into the renal lymphatics or peritubular capillaries. The macula densa is considered a chemoreceptor that responds to chemical changes in Na^+, K^+, and other ionic concentrations. The cells of the afferent arteriole, on the other hand, are considered baroreceptors, responding primarily to changes in the blood pressure within the afferent arteriole. Of course, this blood pressure may reflect the systemic blood pressure.

Some physiologists argue that the role of the macula densa is important mainly for regulation of *intrarenal* renin, which would affect the GFR and RBF through production of angiotensin within the kidney itself. Angiotensin is a vasoconstricting substance, and evidence for its intrarenal production exists. It would exert its effect through vascular changes in the arterioles of the glomerulus. Such an action might be the basis of renal autoregulation. In addition, renin release would have systemic effects, as outlined in Fig. 4-5. It is seen that renin is really an enzyme that

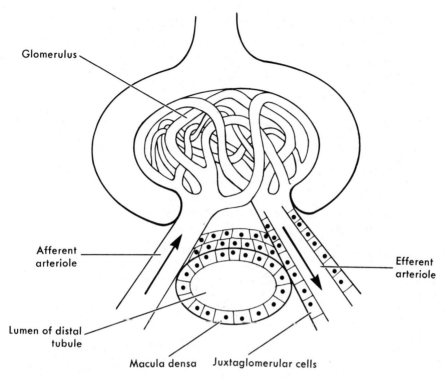

Fig. 4-6. Juxtaglomerular apparatus: specialized renal cells that secrete renin. (From Groër, M. E., and Shekleton, M. E.: Basic pathophysiology: a conceptual approach, St. Louis, 1979, The C. V. Mosby Co.)

causes the enzymatic conversion of renin substrate to angiotensin I. Renin substrate is normally present in an inactive state in the blood, and its production is stimulated by estrogenic compounds. Angiotensin I is present only briefly in the blood and is acted on by converting enzyme, which is produced and active in the lung tissue and is also present in a limited quantity in the blood. Converting enzyme causes angiotensin I to be converted to angiotensin II, a potent vasoconstricting agent that is rapidly removed from the blood by the action of angiotensinases. Thus its vasopressor action is of very short duration. The major effect of angiotensin II is to stimulate the cells of the zona glomerulosa of the adrenal cortex to release aldosterone. This hormone has one major action but many target tissues. Its effect is to increase Na^+ reabsorption and thus conserve total body Na^+. Although its major target organ is the kidney, aldosterone has been shown to increase Na^+ reabsorption in the sweat

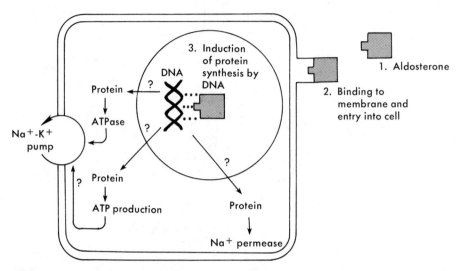

Fig. 4-7. Theoretic mechanisms of aldosterone-induced protein synthesis by renal tubular cells.

glands, gastrointestinal tract, and other tissues. The mechanism of action of aldosterone is presently unknown, although several theories of action exist and are outlined in Fig. 4-7. Aldosterone has no effect on PCT Na^+ reabsorption but acts on the distal nephron, the DCT, and the collecting ducts to increase Na^+ reabsorption and conversely to increase K^+ and H^+ secretion. The action of aldosterone appears to be through entry into the cell and subsequent attachment to a cytoplasmic receptor molecule. The complex thus formed is believed to then move into the nucleus and act on the DNA, causing it to direct the synthesis of a particular protein or proteins. The controversy over aldosterone is not about whether new protein synthesis results when aldosterone enters the nephron cells but rather about what kinds of proteins are produced. Fig. 4-7 shows the three postulated proteins that may be stimulated by aldosterone. One speculation is that a protein is formed which stimulates the formation of ATP, the fuel required for the Na^+ pump. It has also been suggested that ATPase is produced through aldosterone and that the availability of specific ATPase involved in Na^+ pumping would increase transport sites or transport efficiency. The third hypothesis is that a specific Na^+ permease is produced by aldosterone-stimulated DNA. This protein would act at the membrane to increase the membrane's permeability for Na^+ and thereby cause increased diffusion from the tubular filtrate into the cells. The Na^+ pump would respond to the increased cellular concentration by increase activity. All these suggestions have some experimental proof to support them.

Aldosterone's major action is on Na^+ reabsorption. However, it is important to point out that other actions may also be caused by the Na^+ effect. Most of the water reabsorption in the tubules is osmotic in nature. Therefore Na^+ reabsorption results in osmotic water movement out of the luminal fluid, followed by isotonic expansion of the ECF, which is transient in nature in case of aldosterone excess. Conversely, the result of an adrenalectomy is a dramatic loss of Na^+ and water through the urine. Aldosterone also stimulates K^+ secretion, since Na^+ reabsorption occurs mainly through a linked pump. In fact, excessive serum K^+ can directly stimulate aldosterone release from the adrenal cortex without the mediation of the renin-angiotensin mechanism. Excessive amounts of aldosterone result in hypokalemia. Aldosterone also affects acid-base balance, since it causes K^+ secretion, and excesses result in hypokalemia. Hypokalemia causes H^+ to substitute for K^+ on the Na^+-K^+ renal pump. Thus excess H^+ is lost, resulting in a state of metabolic alkalosis.

Water reabsorption. Although water reabsorption is controlled in large part by the amount of sodium reabsorption, there is another regulatory system that functions in the distal nephron. The antidiuretic hormone (ADH) acts on the collecting ducts of certain nephrons, the juxtamedullary nephrons, to increase the water permeability of the luminal cells. The juxtamedullary nephrons constitute about 20% of the total nephrons and are characterized by very long loops of Henle, which dip down deep into the renal medulla. ADH acts to increase water reabsorption from the tubular filtrate in these nephrons. This increase causes less urine to be excreted and thus has an antidiuretic effect. In the absence of ADH, large amounts of urine would be lost every day. There is, in fact, a condition, diabetes insipidus, characterized by the excretion of up to nearly 3 liters of dilute urine every day. This condition often arises as the result of a tumor or traumatic injury to the hypothalamic area, which is responsible for production and release of ADH. Fig. 4-8 describes the location of this center, the manner of storage of hormone in the neurohypophysis, and the ways in which its release is stimulated. Of course, the major mechanism for ADH release is an increase in plasma osmolarity. It is believed that the cells of the supraoptic and paraventriculur nuclei respond osmotically to changes in plasma osmolarity; thus the cells shrink when a hypertonic plasma is present. This stimulates production of ADH, which increases water reabsorption and subsequently decreases the

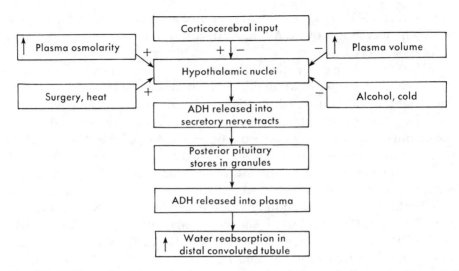

Fig. 4-8. ADH production and release are regulated through plasma volume and plasma osmolarity; increases in plasma volume are inhibitory, and decreases are stimulatory. Increased plasma osmolarity will stimulate production, and decreased osmolarity inhibits ADH. Other inputs are also indicated.

plasma osmolarity, as well as expands the ECF. Another stimulus to ADH is believed to be the actual blood volume. True volume receptors have as yet not been identified, but their existence seems likely. Mechanisms of control of ADH release were reviewed in Chapter 2, and the reader is referred to this discussion as an introduction to the following description of ADH action on the kidneys.

Before detailing the action of ADH on the collecting ducts, we will review the general mechanisms of water reabsorption along the length of the nephron. There is an obligatory amount of water that must be passed in the urine each day: it is the volume needed to dissolve the waste products that must be excreted. The less water that is actually excreted, the greater will be the osmolarity and specific gravity of the urine. Conversely, greater water loss is associated with a dilute urine of low specific gravity and osmolarity. Table 4-1 shows the relationship of specific gravity to osmolarity. Specific gravity is conveniently measured with a urinometer, but urine osmolarity requires more complicated instrumentation.

The range of specific gravity in human urine is from 1.003 to 1.030; the average value is 1.010. The minimum urine output is 500 ml/24 hr—the obligatory volume. This, then, is the minimum amount of water that

Table 4-1. Relationship of specific gravity to osmolarity

Specific gravity	Osmolarity (mOsm/liter)
1.005	200
1.007	300
1.010	400
1.020	800
1.030	1200
1.035	1400

will hold the waste products of metabolism and is thus a reflection of the maximum concentrating ability of the kidneys. The specific gravity of this urine is 1.032, and it contains 700 mOsm. Since the normal urine output is 1 ml/min, urine will normally be excreted in a volume of 1440 ml/24 hr. This urine contains the 700 mOsm that must be excreted daily and therefore has an osmolarity of nearly *490 mOsm*. The range of normal urine osmolarity is 200 to 1200 mOsm/24 hr. When urine osmolarity reaches the maximum concentration of 1400 mOsm/liter, the urine is five times more concentrated than plasma, which is approximately 300 mOsm/liter. The amount of waste products that must be excreted daily can be reduced to a low of 200 mOsm if an individual is on a diet containing no protein or fat and only enough glucose to meet caloric needs. The waste products that are usually excreted are largely nitrogenous, and therefore the elimination of dietary protein decreases these wastes. When the number of milliosmoles produced by metabolism is reduced to only 200 mOsm, the urine water loss can then be decreased to an obligatory volume of 150 ml! This phenomenon will provide some of the rationale for the dietary treatment of individuals with acute renal failure.

Water is reabsorbed along the length of the tubule, and its mechanism of reabsorption is osmotic in nature. Therefore, as other osmotically active substances are reabsorbed, water will osmose with them to maintain the osmolarity of the tubular cells and interstitium. This mechanism of course requires that the tubular epithelium be freely permeable to water throughout. In fact, some areas of the nephron are impermeable to water. The most significant area is the ascending limbs of the juxtamedullary nephrons. The water permeability of the DCT, and especially of the collecting duct, is adjusted by the hormone ADH. These segments of the nephron are usually considered only slightly permeable to water, but since ADH increases the permeability significantly, more water will move through the tubular epithelium of the collecting ducts and thus will be absorbed into the capillary blood. ADH is a hormone that is continuously released, and therefore the normal physiology of the collecting duct is toward antidiuresis. When ADH is absent, the urine volume increases dramatically.

Countercurrent exchange. To better appreciate how ADH regulates urine volume and water reabsorption, one must understand the *countercurrent osmotic multiplier* function of the juxtamedullary nephrons. It is through the anatomy and physiology of these nephrons that water balance is ultimately achieved. Fig. 4-9 diagrams the anatomy of such a nephron in schematic manner. Notice that the loop of Henle is very long as compared to a cortical nephron. Further, the peritubular capillary system (the vasa recta) of these nephrons consists of long vessels that dip deep into the medulla of the kidney, along with the loops of Henle. Fluid flows

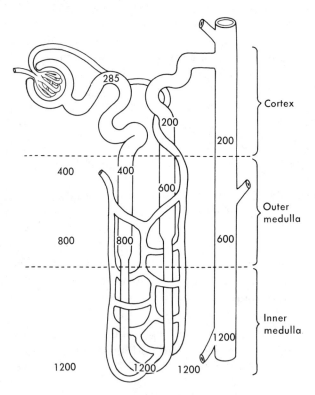

Fig. 4-9. Juxtamedullary nephron.

in both the loops of Henle and the vasa recta in two opposing directions (i.e., in a countercurrent manner). Fluid flows down the descending limbs, through hairpin turns, and up into the ascending limbs. The same pattern of blood flow occurs in the capillaries.

The countercurrent principle has long been used to efficiently heat water in pipes. Water that moves in a countercurrent direction through pipe bent into a loop can be heated by applying a heater to the hairpin loop. The water in each limb then exchanges heat with the water in the other limb, and the overall temperature of the water in the pipe is much higher than it would be if water were heated in a straight-pipe system. The effect is a multiplier one.

A similar multiplier effect occurs in the kidney, but the osmotic pressure of the fluid in the nephron is the factor that is multiplied. It is through an exchange of water and osmotic particles that osmolarity of the fluid in the tubule and renal interstitium, as well as in the capillaries, is altered. Fig. 4-10 illustrates the mechanism of countercurrent exchange in the kidney. Notice that the osmolarity of the fluid entering the descending limb of the loop of Henle is about 285 mOsm. This is very close to the osmolarity of plasma and is caused by the isosmotic reabsorption of water and solutes in the DCT; thus osmolarity is not altered. As the fluid moves down the descending limb, the osmolarity changes drastically, and at the tip of the loop of Henle the osmolarity is very high, about 1200 mOsm. Recall that this osmolarity is about the greatest osmolarity of urine that the kidney can elaborate. As the filtrate moves up into the ascending limb, the osmolarity decreases markedly, and as it moves into the DCT, it is hypotonic to plasma, having an osmolarity of 200 mOsm. The osmolarity changes again as the fluid moves into the collecting duct, from 200 mOsm to as high as 1200 mOsm when ADH is present. Notice that urine having an osmolarity of 200 mOsm is the most dilute urine that the kidney normally makes, as shown in Table 4-1. However, a value of less than 30 mOsm is theoretically possible in the complete absence of ADH. The net effect of osmotic changes, then, is to produce a gradient of increasingly greater osmolarities through the renal medulla. Let us now examine in detail how countercurrent exchange occurs, and it will become apparent that the action of ADH is to allow the concentration of the urine to be regulated as a function of this osmotic gradient produced by the countercurrent osmotic multiplier.

A major key to understanding this mechanism is to note the differential permeabilities of the segments of the nephron to water and sodium. It

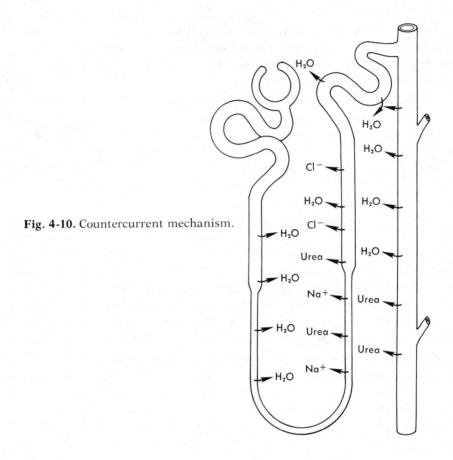

Fig. 4-10. Countercurrent mechanism.

is believed that the descending limb is highly permeable to water but is not permeable to such solutes as sodium and urea. At the beginning of the descending limb, the fluid in the nephron is isosmotic with the fluid in the interstitium, but as the fluid in the descending limb moves through this portion, the water osmoses out of the luminal membrane and into the interstitium. Since no sodium moves out through the membrane, the fluid that is left behind becomes increasingly hypertonic. The osmotic movement of water occurs in response to an increasingly higher concentration of solute within the interstitium caused by movement of sodium, chloride, and urea out of the water-impermeable ascending limb. Thus the filtrate in both the descending and ascending limbs becomes more concentrated. The fluid in the interstitium also becomes progressively more hypertonic, and the greatest hypertonicity is reached at the tip of the loop of Henle. Notice that as the fluid moves into the thick portion of the ascending limb, the osmolarity becomes progressively less, since solute continues to move out of the tubule. Then, as the fluid moves into the DCT and collecting duct, the osmolarity again begins to change. The osmolarity of the fluid in the collecting duct reflects the osmolarity of the medullary interstitium in the presence of ADH. Two phenomena of importance to urine-concentrating ability occur in the collecting duct. The first is the differential permeability of the collecting duct to urea. In the outer medulla the collecting duct is impermeable to urea, and its water permeability depends on the presence of ADH. When ADH is present, water moves into the interstitium and leaves behind a highly concentrated filtrate with a large amount of urea. In the inner medulla the tubular epithelium is permeable to urea and also to water in the presence of ADH. The urea diffuses into the interstitium and helps to maintain the hypertonicity of the medullary interstitium, which is a necessity for countercurrent multiplication. Furthermore, as water diffuses into the interstitium when ADH is present, the urine left behind is concentrated. Urine formed in the collecting ducts of the inner medulla is as dilute or concentrated as it will ever be and is basically ready to be excreted.

Adequate concentrating ability of the kidney depends not only on countercurrent exchange but on the hypertonicity of the interstitium, which must be maintained so that the action of ADH will allow the urine to come into osmotic equilibrium with the interstitium. Recall that as the filtrate is being reabsorbed along the length of the nephron, large amounts of water are moving into the capillary blood. If the capillary blood flow were very rapid, it would quickly wash out the osmotic gradient in the medulla. Therefore another requirement of the countercurrent mechanism is that capillary blood flow be sluggish. Not only do the anatomy and physiology of the vasa recta allow blood to move slowly through the capillary network, but the vasa recta themselves participate in countercurrent exchange. Notice that the vasa recta form hairpin loops characterized by the countercurrent flow of the capillary blood. There is a typical countercurrent exchange across the endothelial walls of these vessels. Water moves out of the descending portions of the vasa recta in response to osmotic gradients, and solutes move out of the ascending portions in response to diffusion gradients. The solutes diffuse back into the descending portions, and the water osmoses back into the ascending portions. This recirculation of water and solutes produces a high osmolarity at the hairpin loop and a reflection of the normal medullary interstitial gradient from inner medulla to outer medulla.

SECRETION

The process of secretion has been mentioned several times because it does not occur in isolation from the other physiologic processes involved in urine formation. The phenomenon is basically a process by which substances that have not been filtered, or that have been filtered only in small amounts, are added into the tubular filtrate along the length of the nephron so that they can be excreted from the body. Most secretion involves active transport in the PCT and is exemplified by the linked Na^+-H^+ pump in the tubule. Sodium reabsorption is linked to either H^+ or K^+ secretion. Other substances that are secreted include ammonia; creatinine; a variety of organic bases such as thiamine, choline, and histamine; anions such as sulfates; and a variety of chemicals or drugs. The drugs include *penicillin*, and inhibition of penicillin secretion by *probenecid* will promote the maintenance of high blood levels of penicillin for longer periods of time. The measurement of creatinine clearance by the kidney reflects the ability of the kidney not only to filter but also to secrete. Since secreted, as well as reabsorbed, substances have a T_m, a maximum rate of secretion for each substance can be achieved.

OTHER KIDNEY FUNCTIONS

The kidneys play a major role as a body buffering system contributing to the regulation of acidity of the body fluids. The pH of the ECF and ICF must be carefully maintained. Small variations cause great physiologic effects. Chapter 5 describes the role of hydrogen ions, the regulation of body pH, and the pathophysiologic results of alteration in acid-base balance. Therefore the role of the kidneys and the mechanisms of urine acidification will also be discussed there.

Other kidney functions are being discovered constantly. It is now known that the kidney cells are similar to the liver in their ability to detoxify many substances. The kidney is an endocrine organ also, releasing activated vitamin D, renin, and the hormone erythropoietin. The latter acts on the bone marrow to stimulate erythropoiesis, and therefore a person with renal disease frequently is anemic. An additional function of the kidney is amino acid oxidation and deamination, a function that allows maintenance of protein metabolism and the common metabolic pool.

The point should be made that normal kidney function is not possible if the urination mechanism is not intact. Normal urinary tract structure and normal physiology of the micturition reflex are necessary. If, for example, an obstruction develops in the ureters, bladder, or urethra, kidney function could be compromised by the increasing backward pressure that would result. As hydrostatic pressure within the collecting ducts and renal tubules increased, a continuously decreasing filtration force would be generated within the glomerulus, and renal shutdown might result. Therefore, whenever the kidney's maintenance of fluid, electrolyte, or pH balance is considered, the entire urinary apparatus must be considered as well. A patient may have a small volume of urine because of dehydration or impending shock, but obstructive urinary tract disease or trauma might also produce the same symptoms. Thus a complete assessment of the patient is obviously required.

The discussion of renal function will be completed with a description of the condition of renal failure, including the manifestations of the condition and the nursing assessments.

ACUTE RENAL FAILURE

Renal function may suddenly cease when the kidneys become ischemic. Ischemia results in death, or necrosis, of the tubular cells, and thus the processes of filtration, reabsorption, and secretion may all become impaired. Some possible causes of renal ischemia include poisons such as heavy metals, obstructions such as that caused by clumps of immune complexes or hemagglutinated cells, infection (e.g., glomerulonephritis), and loss of blood supply caused by prolonged vasoconstriction. It is important to be aware of the latter possibility whenever a patient is in any form of shock accompanied by widespread sympathetic nervous system activation. Recall that the sympathetic nerves constrict the afferent arteriole, reducing RBF and GFR. Decreasing urinary output in the patient in shock is a sign of impending renal failure. Acute renal failure is characterized by urine production of less than 400 ml/24 hr. Normal urine output is 1 ml/min, or 60 ml/hr. This latter value should be remembered so that changes become immediately apparent to the nurse who is caring for a patient with possible alterations in kidney funciton. Complete anuria is not often present, but oliguria can be present for up to 3 weeks. If recovery occurs, the kidneys begin to function by producing a very dilute urine during the early and late portions of the diuretic phase. The reabsorptive and secretory mechanisms of the tubules are not efficient at this time. The actual diuresis that occurs during this phase of recovery reflects an increased GFR without an accompanying increase in reabsorption. As the renal tubular epithelium grows and matures in function, reabsorption and secretion begin to function, and the patient may experience a period of recovery lasting a year or more. Total recovery is possible after acute renal failure. It depends in large part on the length of the period of ischemia, the degree and extent of the tubular necrosis, and the recovery capacity of the individual. An elderly person, for example, is not likely to ever recover completely from an episode of acute renal failure.

During the acute phase of this disease process, the loss of normal kidney function has dramatic effects on every system of the body. Fluid retention is obviously a great problem, since the normal major water excretory route is not present. The volume regulation that is necessary to adjust output with intake is largely renal. Other water loss routes do attempt to compensate by increasing their output, but the water load that these routes can handle is much less than that required. Therefore a major form of treatment of patients in acute renal failure is fluid restriction. However, even with water restriction, patients with acute renal failure are experiencing great stress and are often in a state of hypermetabolism. The water of oxidation produced as a by-product of metabolism is increased, and this water load is additive with the fluids ingested in the diet. The fluid intake depends on several factors but is almost always less than 1 liter/24 hr and can be as little as 400 ml/24 hr in the severely stressed patient.

Another great problem in acute renal failure is the accumulation of waste products normally excreted by the kidneys. Notable among these products are nitrogenous wastes and various acids such as sulfuric acid, phosphoric acid, and by-products of incomplete fat metabolism. Normally 16 gm of nitrogenous wastes is produced daily. This amount can be reduced to less than 5 gm/24 hr if a protein-free diet is consumed. Muscle metabolism can also be decreased by limitation of muscular activity. The effects of these restrictions are to decrease the load on the kidneys and reduce the state of uremia that exists in acute renal failure. Uremia is the condition describing the syndrome produced by accumulation of nitrogenous wastes in the blood. Most systems of the body are affected in some way by these wastes and by the loss of kidney function. A decrease in nervous conduction, alterations in the central nervous system leading to convulsions, and bizarre behavior are typical. The skin becomes highly pruritic and sometimes hyperpigmented. Because the gastrointestinal tract often becomes involved, the patient complains of nausea, vomiting, and diarrhea. There may be cardiac failure and hypertension, as well as generalized muscle wasting and weakness. Most of the other systems are involved either directly or indirectly. The waste products present in the blood are measured by a test, known as the BUN test, that measures nitrogen balance. Another parameter measured is the nonprotein nitrogen (NPN), which reflects uric acid, urea, and creatinine. Both of these values increase dramatically in acute renal failure.

The third major area of concern in the patient with acute renal failure is acidosis and electrolyte imbalance. Acidosis results from both the accumulation of acid wastes and an inability of the kidneys to secrete H^+. Recall that there is a dilutive effect on the electrolytes present in the ECF if edema is present. Increases or decreases in body fluid electrolyte concentrations should thus be assessed with this effect in mind. Many patients will be hyponatremic, largely as the result of the dilutive effects on the serum sodium. The total body sodium, on the other hand, may actually be increased. In acute renal failure, calcium and phosphate balance is usually disturbed (hypocalcemia and hyperphosphaturia), as discussed in Chapter 9. The electrolyte imbalance with the most serious consequences is hyperkalemia, because of the loss of renal regulation of the serum concentration of K^+. (The pathophysiologic disturbances caused by hyperkalemia are described in detail in Chapter 8.) Briefly, excess ECF K^+ results in increased nervous system irritability, muscle weakness, and cardiac conduction abnormalities.

An additional problem in patients with acute renal failure is altered osmotic pressure of the ECF because of accumulated wastes. The result is osmosis of water into the ECF and consequent cellular dehydration. Of course, a wide variety of physiologic disturbances ensue, as well as stimulation of thirst, a need that must be left unmet in acute renal failure.

Treatment

The kidneys are necessary for survival. Loss of kidney function often necessitates dialysis of the wastes and electrolytes through a variety of techniques during the early stage of renal shutdown. Other approaches to treatment of acute renal failure include dietary therapy. The diet should be high in carbohydrates (150 gm/24 hr) and low in proteins for reasons discussed earlier in this chapter. The net effect of this diet is to decrease the accumulation of nitrogenous waste in the blood. Furthermore, a sodium and potassium restriction and a total fluid restriction are usually necessary; the amount of ingested water allowed is based on losses of water from the available water loss compartments. The intake and output of patients with acute renal failure must be recorded diligently, and their weight is also carefully measured every day. Pharmacologic treatment of acute renal failure is limited, but occasionally the blood of patients with severe acidosis will require alkalinization. Other drugs used include antibiotics, digitalis, exchange resins, antiemetics, and IV fluids. Some patients will be incapacitated by the severity of the anemia that usually develops as the result of decreased erythropoietin levels. Patients may also suffer from thrombocytopenia (a decrease in circulating platelets), which enhances bleeding, bruising, and formation of petechiae. Such patients may require whole blood or platelet transfusions, which have a short-term benefit. Red blood cell survival is limited in patients with uremia, whether the cells are transfused or are the endogenously produced erythrocytes.

Fluid overload may result in hypertension and congestive heart failure, and digitalis is often administered.

When and if the patient enters the early diuretic phase of acute renal failure, the needs and problems change. In this situation there is a fluid deficit that can quickly develop because of the diuresis of large amounts of dilute urine. The patient may lose salt and water, which must be replaced to maintain the steady state. Thus the previously severely restricted patient must now have increased oral or IV fluid and salt intake. The gradual recovery of the ability of the tubules to concentrate the urine eventually returns urinary output to normal, although this process may take many months. There is a possibility that chronic renal failure will develop after the acute phase, and some patients do not recover from acute renal failure because of the complications of bleeding, infection, and fluid, electrolyte, and acid-base disturbances.

Signs and symptoms

The patient in acute renal failure has a wide variety of possible signs and symptoms. Most patients feel weak and complain of malaise, loss of appetite, an unpleasant taste in the mouth, and fatigue. Pruritus may be severe, and the crystals of urea may actually be visible on the skin surface (uremic frost). Petechiae and bruising are often marked, and there is the general pallor that accompanies anemia. Patients in severe hypervolemia may develop the signs and symptoms of heart failure and pulmonary edema. Hypertension is usually present, and the diastolic pressure is particularly high in some patients. There may or may not be obvious interstitial edema and ascites in the patient with cardiac complications. Signs of secondary infection may be additive with the renal-related pathology, since infection is common and carries a grave prognosis. The patient may be semicomatose and in all cases will have some degree of impairment of neurologic function because of uremia, hyperkalemia, hypervolemia, hypernatremia, or a combination of these problems. The possibility of hypocalcemia's contributing to the signs and symptoms should also be considered. Many patients will have disruptions of the gastrointestinal functioning, such as nausea, vomiting, and diarrhea. An occasional patient will develop pancreatitis as a result of obstruction of the pancreatic ducts with uremic waste products.

Nursing care and physical assessment of the patient in acute renal failure

The nursing care of the patient in acute renal failure is a critical factor in the patient's eventual prognosis. Avoidance of infection, for example, is largely a nursing responsibility. The patient is greatly at risk for infection, which in fact is the most common cause of death. Scrupulous hygienic measures directed toward avoidance of pathogens are thus required. Other nursing strategies designed to increase the coping defenses of the patient are as important. For example, coughing and deep breathing, frequent turning, and encouragement of full respiratory excursion through any other acceptable means will increase the ability of the patient to cope with respiratory pathogens. Attention to catheters and other portals of entry should also be part of the nursing care plan. For some patients, reverse isolation may be required, to prevent the introduction of common hospital organisms into the patient's environment. Since many of the early signs of infection may be confused with the uremia-related problems, the assessment of the patient must be constant and record keeping continuous. Primary nursing is an ideal approach for a patient with critical illness of this nature, in which slight observable changes may indicate potentially great physiologic disruptions.

The safety of the environment must be a factor in nursing care, not only to prevent infection, but also to decrease the chance of injury to a patient with compromised coagulation. Comfort of the patient who is weak or sometimes even semicomatose obviously is also considered by the nurse who is planning care.

Planning a diet with the dietitian and patient may be a nursing responsibility. A diet low in salt, potassium, and protein and high in calories is ideal. It must be combined, however, with fluid restriction. Because of the gastrointestinal dysfunction, the patient may need to be on a liquid diet, but the fluid status usually precludes it. Nevertheless, the patient's nutritional integrity plays a major role in immunocompetence and nitrogen balance and therefore affects the recovery from the acute disease process. Some patients may need IV feeding or even hyperalimentation, but care must be taken not to cause fluid overload or increased osmotic

Table 4-2. Physical assessment and nursing care of the patient in acute renal failure

System	Problems	Physical assessment	Nursing strategies
Integumentary	Uremic frost; pruritus; edema; pallor; infection; petechiae and ecchymoses	Daily inspection of the skin; palpation for skin turgor and presence of pitting	Skin care; frequent sponging of the skin; antipruritic drugs
Head, eyes, ears, nose, throat	Headache; bleeding into gums; epistaxis; blurred vision caused by hypertension; halitosis; infection	Inspection of the nose, mouth, and throat; ophthalmoscopic examination of the fundi; inspection for signs of infection	Mouth care; avoidance of trauma to nose and mouth; dimly lighted room
Cardiovascular	Hypertension, particularly diastolic; congestive heart failure; pulmonary edema; cardiac arrhythmias	Auscultation for decreased heart sounds, abnormalities in rhythm, rales, rhonchi, and other adventitial sounds; palpation of the peripheral pulses	Daily weights; strict intake and output; salt and fluid restriction; limited exercise; cardiac monitoring; vital signs as necessary
Respiratory	Depressed cough and creased respiratory effort because of fatigue, coma, etc; pulmonary edema; accumulation of secretions because of immobility; increased respiratory rate because of metabolic acidosis	Inspection of respiratory effort; auscultation of the lungs; percussion of the thorax for accumulation of fluid, diaphragmatic excursion; palpation for tactile fremitus	Vital signs as necessary; available O_2 and suction; encouragement of turning, coughing, deep breathing
Hematopoietic	Decreased platelet, white blood cell, and erythrocyte counts, with pallor, fatigue, and susceptibility to bruising	Inspection of skin and mucous membranes	Avoidance of pathogens, trauma, and stress; provision of stable environmental temperature; conservation of patient's energies
Musculoskeletal	Decreased muscle strength; muscle twitching; restless leg syndrome	Inspection of muscle mass; palpation of muscle strength; range of motion of joints; palpation of bones for fractures, tender areas	Provision of safe environment; limited exercise to decrease muscle protein catabolism

Table 4-2. Physical assessment and nursing care of the patient in acute renal failure—cont'd

System	Problems	Physical assessment	Nursing strategies
Neurologic	Increased irritability caused by hyper-kalemia, hypocal-cemia; mental confusion, peripheral sensory disturbances; eventual coma	Complete neurologic examination including evaluation of deep tendon reflexes and sensory, motor, and cortical function	Provision of a quiet, safe environment; orientation to time, place, person, etc.; frequent assessment of neurologic integrity
Renal	Anuria or oliguria with production of urine of low specific gravity; acidosis (metabolic); hyperkalemia, hypernatremia, hypocalcemia, hyperphosphatemia; azotemia	Palpation of kidneys; determination of tenderness of costovertebral angle; inspection of urinary stream; assessment of electrolyte disturbances as described in Chapter 5	Ongoing evaluation of urine specific gravity; fluid restriction as appropriate to output; input and output; daily weights; dietary restrictions
Gastrointestinal	Thirst; nausea; vomiting; diarrhea; ascites; signs and symptoms of pancreatitis	Palpation of abdomen for tenderness, masses; auscultation of bowel sounds; percussion of abdomen for shifting dullness	Food provided in attractive manner; antiemetics as ordered; mouth care; observation of stools; high-calorie liquids; patient participation in planning allotment of fluids

effects on the already hyperosmolar plasma. Because of the altered renal metabolism and decreased excretory ability, some drugs are neither detoxified nor excreted well, and the possibility of addictive effects and drug interactions must be considered.

The range of nursing assessments in the care of this patient is extremely wide. Assessment must be thorough, systematic, and ongoing. The patient's history is necessary in planning appropriate care. Specific aspects of the nursing history should include not only those factors that may have contributed to the disease but also those activities of daily living that are characteristic of the patient. Food likes and dislikes, activity and exercise levels, occupation, recreational pursuits, and habits should be part of the nurse's data base in planning holistic care.

The physical assessment of the patient in acute renal failure is complex and should be part of every nurse's initial and cumulative collection of data as the care plan is developed. Table 4-2 lists the systematic physical assessment of the patient. The individual nurse must modify the suggested approach as the patient's condition and problems dictate.

CASE STUDY

This case study shows the progression of acute glomerulonephritis into acute and then chronic disease, ending with renal failure.

HISTORY

A 22-year-old woman entered the hospital because she had "passed tea-colored urine for 2 days." During the previous week she had noticed increasing puffiness of her hands and face, fatigue, anorexia, and a persistent headache. She recalled having had a sore throat about a month before admission.

PHYSICAL EXAMINATION

Examination in the hospital produced the following findings:
Weight: 68 kg
Blood pressure: 180/100
Vital signs: 100/80/20
Laboratory data:
   BUN: 30 mg/dl
   GFR: 40 ml/min
   Hematocrit: 35%
   Hemoglobin: 10.5 gm/dl
   Urinalysis:
      Color: red
      Specific gravity: 1.020
      pH: 6
      Glucose, ketones: negative
      Sediment: many red cells, white cells, casts
The patient was a slightly obese woman in no acute distress. Her physical examination was within normal limits except for the following:
   Extremities: pitting edema of hands and feet, cold to touch
   Chest: negative except for tenderness of costovertebral angle (CVA) on both right and left sides
   Abdomen: pain during deep palpation of both right and left kidneys
   Neurologic findings: mild hyperreflexia and slight tremor of hands

HOSPITAL COURSE. The diagnosis was acute glomerulonephritis, and the patient recovered, being discharged in 3 weeks. After 4 months her GFR was 120 ml/min and her BUN level was 10.

She did well until 2 years later, when she developed marked generalized edema and was rehospitalized. Her face, limbs, and abdomen were massively swollen (edema). Blood pressure was 200/110, GFR was

70 ml/min, and the serum albumin level was 1 gm/dl. The urinalysis showed 3+ albumin. The diagnosis was nephrotic syndrome. The patient continued to have similar episodes for 3 more years, and tests showed gradually decreasing renal function. Seven years after her initial illness she entered the hospital because of confusion, marked fatigue, and anorexia. She appeared at that time to be a wasted, chronically ill woman. Blood pressure was 210/130; weight was 53 kg.

Laboratory results:

Hematocrit: 28%

Hemoglobin: 6 gm/dl

BUN: 140 mg/dl

GFR: 10 ml/min

Urinalysis:

Albumin: 3+

Specific gravity: 1.012

The woman was not able to concentrate her urine, although she was dehydrated. Her BUN level rose to 220 units and her urine output fell to 50 ml/24 hr. On the twelfth hospital day she went into severe acidosis, her potassium level rose dangerously, and she became comatose. She developed pneumonia and died quietly on the twentieth hospital day.

5
Acid-base balance and imbalance

The regulation of the pH of the body fluids is accomplished through many physiologic mechanisms. The importance of maintaining normal pH is dramatically demonstrated by patients with altered plasma pH. The normal range is small, and numerous coping mechanisms must be brought into play to compensate for a change in pH. Even then, tolerance of increased or decreased acidity of the body fluids is limited, and death will result when the pH is significantly altered for a long enough time.

The hydrogen ion concentration (H^+ concentration) influences almost every biochemical reaction that takes place within the body fluids. The pH also has profound effects on lipid integrity and protein bonding and therefore on the structure and function of all membranes. The ability of enzymes to function is greatly altered by a rise or drop in pH; thus normal physiologic processes can occur only when the pH is constant.

The normal physiologic regulation of acid-base balance will be described in this chapter. Pathophysiologic alterations in the acid-base balance and the compensatory mechanisms that operate to maintain this balance will be discussed in detail. The reader will first be introduced to the physiochemistry of the acid-base balance of the blood.

HYDROGEN ION CONCENTRATION (pH)
Units of pH

The term *pH* refers to the negative logarithm of the H^+ concentration. The range of pH is from 1 to 14 units. It is important to appreciate the tremendous change in concentration of H^+ when comparing pH units. Table 5-1 shows the actual concentrations of H^+ and the corresponding pH units.

Table 5-1. Hydrogen ion concentrations and corresponding pH units

H⁺ concentration (gm/liter)	Scientific notation	pH units
0.1	10^{-1}	$-\log 10^{-1} = 1$
0.01	10^{-2}	$-\log 10^{-2} = 2$
0.001	10^{-3}	$-\log 10^{-3} = 3$
0.0001	10^{-4}	$-\log 10^{-4} = 4$
0.00001	10^{-5}	$-\log 10^{-5} = 5$
0.000001	10^{-6}	$-\log 10^{-6} = 6$
0.0000001	10^{-7}	$-\log 10^{-7} = 7$
0.00000001	10^{-8}	$-\log 10^{-8} = 8$
0.000000001	10^{-9}	$-\log 10^{-9} = 9$
0.0000000001	10^{-10}	$-\log 10^{-10} = 10$
0.00000000001	10^{-11}	$-\log 10^{-11} = 11$
0.000000000001	10^{-12}	$-\log 10^{-12} = 12$
0.0000000000001	10^{-13}	$-\log 10^{-13} = 13$
0.00000000000001	10^{-14}	$-\log 10^{-14} = 14$

Using Table 5-1, compute the difference between a pH of 1 and a pH of 7. Although there is a difference of only 6 pH units between these two numbers, the actual amount is 10^5 H⁺ ions, or a 100,000-fold difference. Notice that the table shows a *decrease* in H⁺ concentration as the pH value increases. The reason is that the pH is a *negative* logarithm. Thus, at the lower pH values, greater amounts of H⁺ are present, indicating a more acid solution. Acidity is a measure of the concentration and activity of H⁺. The normal pH of the extracellular fluid is 7.4. This value is slightly more basic than neutral pH, which is 7, and it represents a concentration of 10^{-7} gm/liter of H⁺. The pH of 7 is the pH of water, the chemical formula of which is H_2O. Some dissociation of the molecules of H_2O does occur in the following manner:

$$H : \ddot{O} : H \rightarrow H^+ + OH^-$$

Whenever a molecule of water dissociates, it releases one H⁺ and one hydroxyl ion (OH⁻). These ions are therefore present in water in exactly the same concentration. Since the pH of water is 7, what is the concentration of OH⁻ in water? It must be the same as H⁺, or 10^{-7} gm/liter. Acid solutions have more H⁺ than OH⁻, whereas basic, or alkaline, solutions have less H⁺ than OH⁻. The sum of the OH⁻ concentration and H⁺ concentration must always equal 10^{-14}. This is known as the *ionization constant of water*. Therefore, when OH⁻ is added to an aqueous solution, the excess OH⁻ will remove H⁺ and form water, and the ionization constant of water (i.e., 10^{-14}) must be maintained. The result must be a rise in pH as H^+ is removed to combine with OH^- to form water. The solution becomes alkaline with a pH greater than 7. Addition of a strong base will result in the release of large amounts of OH^- and the subsequent removal from solution of an equivalent number of H^+. Thus the effect on pH is greater than that of a weak base, which only weakly dissociates and therefore removes less H^+.

Measuring pH

The H^+ concentration of a solution can be measured by the use of indicator dyes (e.g., litmus paper) or, in the clinical setting, of a pH meter. This instrument is highly sensitive to small variations in the pH and is very reliable. It is often convenient, however, for the nurse to check the pH of body fluids, such as urine, feces, or emesis, with some form of litmus paper. Thus a supply should be available so that the nurse can assess changes in the patient's body fluid status.

CHEMISTRY OF ACIDS AND BASES

It is important to have a working knowledge of the physical chemistry of acids and bases. Chemists use several definitions of acids, but the Brönsted-Lowry definition is the most useful one in our discussion. This definition of acidity states that an acid releases H^+, and a base is a substance that takes up, or binds, H^+. The more H^+ that an acid releases, the stronger it is. A substance such as HCl is a very strong acid, since it essentially is completely ionized into H^+ and chloride anion (Cl^-). Most acids present in the blood are weak acids, such as phosphoric acid and carbonic acid. These acids do not readily give up their H^+, and a measure of their strength is provided by the numerical value of their pK. The pK is the negative logarithm of the equilibrium constant (K_{eq}). The understanding of acid-base balance in body fluids will be greatly enhanced if the concept of K_{eq} is clear. The K_{eq} describes the rate constant for a reversible chemical reaction at equilibrium. It is specific for each type of chemical reaction. The following equation should be examined:

$$AB \leftrightarrows A + B$$

Notice that this reaction is reversible. Some AB dissociates into A + B, and the reverse also occurs, forming AB. If AB is a strong acid, then it dissociates completely into A and B, and the reverse reaction does not occur. However, a weak acid will dissociate only a little, and the reverse reaction will occur. This extent of dissociation is indicated by the K_{eq} in the following manner:

$$K_{eq} = \frac{A \times B}{AB}$$

At equilibrium the product of $A \times B$, which are the products in the reaction, divided by the product of the reactants (AB, in this case), will equal a specific value, the equilibrium constant (K_{eq}).

By substituting real values for the components of this chemical reaction, we will be able to see how useful the K_{eq} is. If 1 mole of AB is present, and it is a weakly dissociable substance, then at equilibrium the amount of AB present will be 1 mole minus the small amount that has dissociated, which can be called X. Therefore the denominator of the equation above is $1 - X$. The numerator is the product of A and B, which are produced by the dissociation of AB. This small amount is really equal to $X \times X$, or X^2. Thus for the reaction:

$$K_{eq} = \frac{X^2}{1 - X}$$

To simplify the calculation, we may eliminate the calculation of X in the denominator, since it is such a tiny amount of substance and does not decrease the value of 1 very much. Thus the equation becomes:

$$K_{eq} = \frac{X^2}{1}$$

Now it becomes possible to calculate X, since the K_{eq} of various chemical reactions is easily obtained from charts. If this reaction represented the dissociation of acetic acid, and if 1 mole of acetic acid dissociates and the K_{eq} is known to be 1.8×10^{-5}, then:

$$X = \sqrt{1.8 \times 10^{-5}}, \text{ or } 4.24 \times 10^{-3}$$

Now the correct pH of a 1M acetic acid solution can be calculated, since one of the products of the dissociation of acetic acid is H^+ and is therefore present in a concentration of 4.24×10^{-3} moles. Thus pH $= -\log (4.24 \times 10^{-3})$, a value that can be calculated as 2.37.

Further manipulation of the formula for the dissociation of a weak acid yields a derivative formula known as the Henderson-Hasselbalch equation. This equation is also very useful, since it is particularly important in the physiologic determination of pH, based on such things as Pco_2 of the plasma and the amount of bicarbonate available to buffer H^+. A more complete discussion of these effects will follow later, but a more thorough examination of the Henderson-Hasselbalch equation is now required. Notice that if:

$$K_{eq} = \frac{A \times B}{AB}$$

then:

$$A = K_{eq} \frac{AB}{B}$$

Let us assume that AB is a weak acid such as carbonic acid, which dissociates into bicarbonate anion (HCO_3^-) and H^+:

$$H_2CO_3 \rightleftarrows H^+ + HCO_3^-$$

Then A is equal to the concentration of H^+, and B is the concentration of bicarbonate. If this equation is multiplied throughout by a constant, the negative logarithm, it becomes:

$$-\log(H^+) = -\log K_{eq} -\log \frac{(H_2CO_3)}{HCO_3^-}$$

We know that the negative logarithm of the H^+ concentration is called the pH. The negative logarithm of the K_{eq} is called the pK, and if the negative logarithm of acid divided by base is converted to the equivalent positive logarithm of base divided by acid, the final form of the famous equation reads:

$$pH = pK + \log \frac{base}{acid}$$

The base refers to the anion or, more usually, the salt form of the anion, which in this case would be $NaHCO_3$. This equation permits calculation of several factors, depending on what is known about the equation. If pH and pK are known, then the concentration of acid and base present can be calculated. This calculation is very important in acid-base physiology, since the weak acids and their salts in the blood are known as buffers, and their concentrations are critical to their efficacy as buffers. For the carbonic acid–bicarbonate system in the blood plasma, the normal pH of 7.4 and the normal pK of 6.1 mean that the ratio of bicarbonate to carbonic acid is 20:1. For every molecule of carbonic acid that is present, there is one molecule of sodium bicarbonate. Now imagine that the pH of the blood should drop to 7.0. What would be the proportion of bicarbonate to carbonic acid in this case? Using the Henderson-Hasselbalch equation, make this determination. The answer is 8:1. Imagine also what would happen to pH if the ratio of 20:1 should be shifted, for example, by an increase in CO_2 present in the blood or by changes in the amount of available sodium bicarbonate.

BUFFERS

There are several ways in which excessive H^+ or OH^- is removed from the blood if these ions are present through some abnormality in functioning. One method is known as chemical buffering and is the removal of H^+ or OH^- by weak acids and the salts of the weak acids by chemical combinations in the ECF. Buffering is also accomplished through cellular buffering and the respiratory and renal systems, although these mechanisms are much slower than plasma chemical buffering. The various buffer systems and their rates of action are seen in Table 5-2. The respiratory system regulates the acidity of the blood by altering the carbon dioxide that is exhaled versus that retained in the blood. A decrease in the rate and depth of ventilation, for example, will result in less exhalation of CO_2 and an accumulation of this substance in the blood and other body fluids. A rise in CO_2 will increase the acidity of the blood and body fluids, whereas a rapid rate or increased depth of respiration will have the opposite effect and the pH will rise to a more alkaline value. The kidneys regulate pH as well, although their action takes several days before an effect on the pH is observed. For persons with chronic diseases affecting the pH, the kidneys may be the most important regulator of H^+ concentration. The kidneys can affect ECF pH by altering the amount of H^+ or HCO_3^- that is excreted or reabsorbed. The details of urine acidification and bicarbonate reabsorption will be discussed later.

Table 5-2. Rates of buffering by various mechanisms

Mechanism	Rate
Plasma buffering	Instantly
Respiratory buffering	10-30 min
Cellular buffering	2-4 hr
Renal buffering	Hours to several days

Chemical buffers

There are several weak acid–salt systems that are effective buffers of the plasma. The major one is the carbonic acid–bicarbonate system, which was previously mentioned. To understand the biochemistry of buffering in general, let us closely examine this system. The law of mass action applies to all reversible reactions, such as the one below:

$$CO_2 + H_2O \underset{\text{Carbonic anhydrase}}{\rightleftharpoons} H_2CO_3 \rightleftharpoons H^+ + HCO_3^-$$

There are several crucial things to notice when this chemical reaction is examined. First, the formation of carbonic acid by water and CO_2 does not occur readily in body fluids but must be catalyzed by an enzyme, carbonic anhydrase, which exists only intracellularly. Therefore, to form carbonic acid, CO_2 must diffuse into cells from the ECF. The dissociation of carbonic acid also does not occur readily, since this acid is weak. In fact, we saw that at normal body pH the ratio of HCO_3^- to H_2CO_3 is 20 : 1. These reactions can be speeded up, however, by the concentrations of the various reactants and products according to the law of mass action. If there is an increase in H^+ or bicarbonate in the body fluids, the law of mass action tells us that the reaction will be driven to the left, toward the formation of CO_2 and water. Conversely, a drop in H^+ or HCO_3^- causes more H_2CO_3 to dissociate and further drives the combination of CO_2 toward the formation of carbonic acid. The reaction is driven to the right, with the result that the CO_2 will drop in concentration. Most of acid-base physiology can be understood if the above equation is clear to the student and if the student is able to predict the effects of alterations in any of these components on the plasma pH.

A buffer system is able to maintain the pH of the plasma even when strong acid or alkali is added to it. It does so by quickly binding with H^+, which would otherwise reduce the pH, or, in the case of alkali, by releasing H^+ to bind with OH^-. Examine the above reaction once again. If a large amount of H^+ should suddenly be introduced into the plasma, an occurrence that might result from hypoxic accumulation of lactic acid in actively metabolic tissues, H^+ would cause the reaction to be driven to the left by combining HCO_3^- with it to form carbonic acid. Conversely, the addition of OH^- would result in a removal of H^+, which would bind with OH^- to form water, and the drop in H^+ would be balanced by an increased dissociation of carbonic acid to H^+ and HCO_3^-. In both cases the pH would hardly be affected because of the buffering action of the carbonic acid–sodium bicarbonate system. All buffer systems

Table 5-3. Common plasma buffer systems

Physiologic buffer pairs	pK values
Hb/HHb	7.3
$NaHCO_3/H_2CO_3$	6.1
Na_2HPO_4/NaH_2PO_4	6.8

operate best in certain pH ranges and have a certain capacity to buffer. The buffer system best operates when the pH is close to the pK of the weak acid that comprises it. This is the pH at which the acid most readily releases or takes up H^+. Some acids have more than one hydrogen ion that can be released; therefore there is a pK value for each hydrogen ion given up by the acid. Titration of H_3PO_4 with base shows that there are three pK values for this acid and therefore three ranges of pH at which the system effectively buffers. Table 5-3 lists the common buffer systems of the plasma and their respective pK values.

Another important buffer in the blood is the hemoglobin molecule, which can exist as a weak acid (designated HHb). The hemoglobin molecule is of course completely contained within the erythrocytes and therefore is an intracellular buffer. However, its intracellular action has effects on the ECF pH as well. It is important to note that deoxyhemoglobin is a weaker acid than oxyhemoglobin; therefore the venous blood is capable of greater buffer capacity. Deoxyhemoglobin is present in high concentrations in the capillary and venous blood, as cells take up oxygen and release carbon dioxide as waste. Thus, at the tissues, CO_2 dissolves in plasma and diffuses into the erythrocytes in the blood. Since these cells have a very high concentration of carbonic anhydrase, CO_2 is quickly hydrated to form carbonic acid as soon as it enters the cell. This action allows a gradient for diffusion of CO_2 into the cells to be continuously maintained so that it does not accumulate in the plasma. In fact, the CO_2 produced by metabolism is "carried" as bicarbonate. The carbonic acid that forms in the erythrocytes dissociates into H^+ and HCO_3^-. The HCO_3^- diffuses through the red blood cell membrane into the plasma as soon as it forms. To maintain the cellular electrical neutrality, Cl^- moves into the red cell as bicarbonate moves out. This phenomenon is known as the *chloride shift*. The H^+ formed intracellularly is buffered by the deoxyhemoglobin. However, there is a slight drop in pH in cells in the venous blood and an increase in osmotically active particles inside the erythrocytes, causing them to swell slightly in venous blood. Fig. 5-1 diagrams the changes that

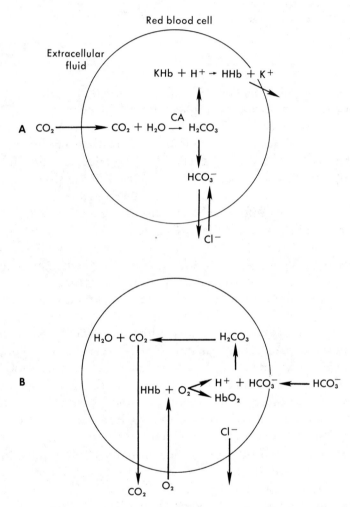

Fig. 5-1. A, Chloride shift and transport of CO_2 into red blood cell at tissue. **B,** Release of CO_2 at lungs. When hemoglobin (Hb) is oxygenated at lungs, it becomes stronger acid, releasing H^+, which results in formation of CO_2. (*CA* = carbonic anhydrase.)

take place in the cell with regard to hemoglobin, Cl^-, CO_2, cations, and pH.

Of course, when the venous blood moves into the pulmonary capillaries, it is exposed to a greater oxygen tension in the alveolar air and a lower CO_2 pressure. The result will be diffusion of oxygen into the plasma and cells and diffusion of CO_2 out of the cells and plasma and into the alveoli. The effects of oxygenation on hemoglobin are profound because the molecule becomes oxyhemoglobin and therefore is a stronger acid. Thus it binds more cations, such as Na^+ and K^+, and releases more H^+. Cl^- diffuses out of the cell to preserve the electrochemical neutrality, and HCO_3^- moves into the erythrocyte, reacts with the liberated H^+, and forms carbonic acid, which dissociates into CO_2 and water. The CO_2 diffuses out of the cells, through the plasma, and into the alveoli. A rapid oxygenation of hemoglobin results in the appropriate exchange of CO_2, which was carried in the plasma as bicarbonate from the blood into the alveoli. Further release of CO_2 from the carbaminohemoglobin form of CO_2 carriage is accomplished at this time, as is also diffusion of any dissolved CO_2. The pH rises as CO_2 is lost from the venous blood, a factor that further aids oxygenation of hemoglobin. Thus the blood leaving the lungs is fully oxygenated and has a lower CO_2 content.

Cellular buffers

It was pointed out earlier that instantaneous buffering is accomplished by the chemical buffers of the blood. Cellular buffering also occurs and is diagramed in Fig. 5-2. Here it can be seen that an excess of H^+ in the ECF creates a gradient for inward diffusion of H^+ into cells. As H^+ is "soaked up" by the cells, other cations are released to maintain electrochemical neutrality. These cations may be either K^+ or Na^+, but since

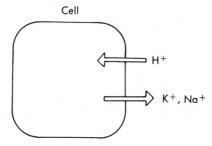

Cell

H^+

K^+, Na^+

Fig. 5-2. As H^+ increases, it diffuses into tissue cells. Diffusion of K^+ and Na^+ out into ECF maintains electrical neutrality.

K^+ is the major intracellular ion, it usually exchanges for H^+. Thus an individual with acidosis may also have an accompanying hyperkalemia, and the reverse is also true (i.e., hypokalemia accompanies alkalosis). The cell proteins attempt to buffer the H^+ as it enters the cell.

Respiratory buffer

Although not acting as rapidly as the plasma buffers or the cells, the respiratory system is nevertheless of great importance in acid-base regulation. The fundamental reason is the control the respiratory system has over the concentration of CO_2 in the blood. As can be seen in the reaction on p. 104, the CO_2 is the major determinant of the speed of the reaction toward the formation of products. As CO_2 accumulates, the reaction is driven toward the right; as it decreases in concentration, the reaction is driven toward the left. A review of the basic components of respiratory physiology that have direct relevance to a discussion of acid-base balance will aid in gaining an understanding of this control.

The carriage of gases in the blood has been discussed. It is obvious that the maintenance of the appropriate partial pressures of these gases is the major function of the respiratory tract. Table 5-4 shows the partial pressures of O_2 and CO_2 in arterial and venous blood in millimeters of mercury.

Both CO_2 and O_2 readily diffuse across all membranes because of their lipid solubility. Their diffusion is regulated by the concentration gradient or, in the case of gases, the pressure gradient. The higher partial pressure of oxygen in the alveolar air results in a rapid diffusion of oxygen into the pulmonary capillary blood. Conversely, the high Pco_2 of venous blood results in a diffusion of CO_2 from the venous blood into the alveolar air. The adequacy of inspiratory and expiratory efforts must be ensured so that the alveolar air partial pressures are maintained. If ventilation becomes inadequate, the Pco_2 of the alveolar air increases and the gradient for CO_2 diffusion into the alveoli subsequently decreases. A rise in

Table 5-4. Gas pressures

	Partial pressure of O_2 (mm Hg)	Partial pressure of CO_2 (mm Hg)
Arterial blood	80-100	40.0
Venous blood	40	46.0
Alveolar air	110	40.0
Dry atmospheric air	160	0.3

blood Pco_2 then follows, with profound effects on acid-base physiology. A rise in H^+ occurs, and a point beyond buffering capacity of the plasma and cells may eventually be reached. At this point the pH of the body fluids would begin to drop dramatically, and a state of respiratory acidosis might ensue. The set of circumstances described above could theoretically happen while a person is in deep sleep. The result would be depression of respiratory movements, a decreased cough reflex, decreased respiratory excursion because of the supine position, and generalized sedation. However, marked acidosis does not occur in deep sleep because of the operation of reflexes that regulate the rate and depth of respiration. Receptors known as the carotid and aortic bodies are very sensitive to Po_2, and when the Po_2 drops, these receptors signal the respiratory centers of the pons and medulla of the brain. A compensatory increase in respiratory rate and depth follows. The respiratory centers are also sensitive to Pco_2 and pH of the plasma, and when pH drops or Pco_2 rises, the increase in respiratory rate and depth results in a greater exhalation of CO_2, with a corresponding drop in Pco_2 in the alveolar air. The converse is true when the pH rises as the result of a drop in CO_2: the respiratory centers are then inhibited, and respiratory rate and depth decrease until an accumulation of CO_2 results in a change of pH toward the normal value. Respiratory control of the pH is the result of constant feedback to the brain centers.

There are many conditions that are basically buffered through respiratory changes. However, when the lungs are diseased, there may be no possibility of the respiratory system's adequately handling the challenge of permanent threats to body fluid pH. The renal system must therefore compensate if survival is to be ensured. The kidneys are well able to perform this buffering function when the cause of the altered pH status is some respiratory disorder of either a primary or a secondary nature.

Renal buffer

The preceding chapter described the normal role of the kidneys in body fluid and electrolyte status but did not fully discuss the acidification of urine or the bicarbonate reabsorption mechanism. They will therefore be described now.

Recall that the urine is formed from a plasma ultrafiltrate and that this ultrafiltrate is very similar in composition to plasma. The pH of the filtrate is about the same as plasma when it is first formed in Bowman's capsule. However, as the filtrate moves through the tubular system, its pH can be changed to a low of 4.5. Thus the pH of the urine is adjusted according to the needs of the body to eliminate H^+ or to reabsorb HCO_3^-. If the urine is to be made acid, there must be secretion of H^+ into the filtrate so that the pH will be lower than that of the ECF. Secretion of H^+ is coupled to the Na^+-K^+ pump reabsorption process. Either K^+ or H^+ can be secreted as Na^+ is being reabsorbed, a phenomenon that appears to be mostly dependent on the ECF concentrations of K^+ and H^+. When H^+ rises, as in acidosis, it will more effectively compete with K^+ on the carrier and therefore will be secreted preferentially over K^+. This increase in H^+, if prolonged, then leads to hyperkalemia, which further contributes to the increased ECF concentration of K^+ that results from cellular buffering.

ACIDIFICATION

Obviously the urine is neither highly acid nor highly alkaline, since the urinary tract would be damaged by such extremes. The amount of H^+ put into the urine each day represents a load of acid produced through metabolism. The amount of acid excreted is much greater than the pH of the urine would suggest at first glance. The reasons are (1) the buffering of H^+ in the tubular filtrate and (2) the actions of other mechanisms, which essentially remove free H^+ and thus maintain normal pH level. The major urinary buffer is phosphate, the acid form of which is monobasic. The dibasic form is filtered at the glomerulus. Ammonia (NH_3) also accepts H^+ and thus removes it from the urine. The sources of these acids that must be excreted are several catabolic processes, including fat and protein breakdown, amino acid metabolism (e.g., cysteine and methionine form sulfuric acid), and the hydrolysis of various esters. The amount of these endogenously produced acids is about 1 mEq/kg/24 hr. The acids produced diffuse into the ECF and must be immediately buffered by HCO_3^- so that the pH is kept constant, according to the reaction on p. 104. Obviously, then, there must be an adequate reserve of bicarbonate available to act in this manner. This reserve is maintained by continuous bicarbonate reabsorption in the proximal convoluted tubule (PCT); thus the plasma concentration in health is approximately 24 mEq/liter. Bicarbonate is filtered at the glomerulus, and the tubular filtrate contains the same bicarbonate concentration as does plasma. However, most of the bicarbonate is reabsorbed in the kidneys, and urine is usually completely free of bicarbonate. There is the possibility of regulation of the amount of bicarbonate that is reabsorbed, however. Since bicarbonate is essentially present to buffer H^+, in states of excess H^+ the kidneys will conserve an equivalent number of HCO_3^- ions beyond the normal. In alkalotic states characterized by high plasma HCO_3^-, excess HCO_3^- is excreted.

Figs. 5-3 to 5-5 diagram the process involved in urine acidification. The first figure shows the formation of *titratable acidity*, that is, NaH_2PO_4. Note that Na^+ exchanges for H^+, as we have previously described. As H^+ moves into the tubular filtrate, it reacts with the phosphoric acid buffer system in the following manner:

$$Na_2HPO_4 + H^+ \rightleftarrows NaH_2PO_4 + Na^+$$

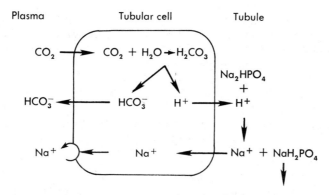

Fig. 5-3. Formation of monobasic phosphoric acid, which is measured as titratable acidity in urine.

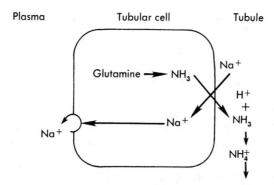

Fig. 5-4. Ammonia reacts with secreted H^+ and neutralizes it, creating ammonium ion, which is excreted. Na^+ can be reabsorbed because electrical neutrality is not disturbed.

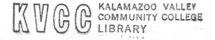

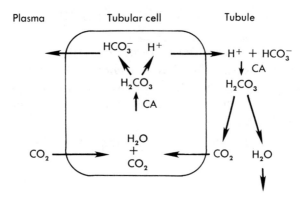

Fig. 5-5. Bicarbonate reabsorption results when carbonic anhydrase *(CA)* inside cell and on tubular luminal membrane catalyzes formation and breakdown of carbonic acid. Note that filtered HCO_3^- is not directly reabsorbed, but no *net* gain or loss of HCO_3^- occurs through this mechanism.

The Na^+ released by the reaction moves into the luminal cell in exchange for H^+, thus maintaining electrical neutrality. The ratio of Na_2HPO_4 to NaH_2PO_4, which is the ratio of salt to acid in this buffer system, is 4:1 at a pH of 7.4, which is the normal pH of plasma and of the glomerular filtrate as well. As acidification occurs, more NaH_2PO_4 forms. This is possible because the pK of this system is 6.8. This pK reflects the ability of Na_2HPO_4 to give up to take up H^+. Thus at an acid pH this buffer is most effective.

Ammonia is also secreted by tubular luminal cells, which break down glutamine to glutamic acid and ammonia. The ammonia is a gas and can very quickly diffuse into the filtrate. Once in the filtrate it combines with available H^+ and forms ammonium ion according to the following reaction:

$$Na^+Cl^- + H^+ + NH_3 \rightarrow NH_4^+Cl^- + Na^+$$

The Na^+ and H^+ exchange for each other as usual.

It is important to understand the source of H^+. Carbon dioxide is present within the ECF and follows a gradient for diffusion into the tubular luminal cells. These cells are among the three cell types containing large amounts of an enzyme, carbonic anhydrase. This enzyme catalyzes the hydration of CO_2 to H_2CO_3, as well as causing the reverse reaction. The CO_2 thus becomes hydrated inside the cells, and then the H_2CO_3 dissociates somewhat into H^+ and HCO_3^-. According to the law of mass

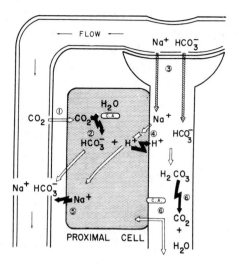

Fig. 5-6. Model of bicarbonate reabsorption in proximal tubule. *1,* Carbon dioxide enters cell, where it is converted to H^+ and bicarbonate in presence of carbonic anhydrase, *2.* Sodium and bicarbonate enter tubule by filtration, *3,* and sodium is exchanged for hydrogen, *4.* Sodium so entering cell is removed on capillary surface by sodium pump, *5,* and bicarbonate in tubule fluid is rapidly converted to carbon dioxide and water by carbonic anhydrase in brush border, *6.* (From Bauman, J. W., Jr., and Chinard, F. P.: Renal function: physiological and medical aspects, St. Louis, 1975, The C. V. Mosby Co.)

action, this latter reaction continues only if H^+ and HCO_3^- leave the cell. The mechanisms of H^+ secretion into the tubular filtrate and HCO_3^- reabsorption are tied together in this mechanism, which allows continuous dissociation of carbonic acid. Fig. 5-6 illustrates the exchange of H^+ for Na^+ and the movement of H^+ into the filtrate. The H^+ may be buffered by the phosphoric acid system or by ammonia, as just described. Another possibility is for the H^+ to combine with filtered HCO_3^-, causing H_2CO_3 to form. Facing the lumen of the PCT is a cellular brush border that contains a high concentration of carbonic anhydrase. Therefore the carbonic acid will dissociate into CO_2 and H_2O, and the CO_2 will then diffuse into the tubular luminal cell. It is important to note that the result is the generation of HCO_3^- *inside* the cell and the subsequent diffusion of HCO_3^- into the plasma. The HCO_3^- is more or less equivalent to the one that was filtered and trapped in the tubular filtrate. Since HCO_3^- cannot pass through the impermeable luminal membrane, the mechanism of reabsorption is indirect. The net result of the process is reabsorption of bicarbonate and secretion of H$^+$ into the filtrate. In a sense the HCO$_3^-$ reabsorbed in this manner maintains the body's reserves of bicarbonate and replaces those ions that were used to buffer the daily H$^+$ load produced endogenously by metabolism.

When excess bicarbonate reabsorption above this basal level is required, the H$^+$ formed by the intracellular hydration of CO$_2$ (the source of which, this time, is only the ECF and not the tubular filtrate) is secreted into the filtrate. There it is buffered and excreted. In this way there is one HCO$_3^-$ reabsorbed that is essentially an extra ion and does not replace the HCO$_3^-$ used to buffer the daily acid load.

ALTERATIONS IN ACID-BASE BALANCE

Before the various disruptions that can occur in acid-base balance are described, let us review the Henderson-Hasselbalch equation once again:

$$pH = pK + \log \frac{base}{acid}$$

The bicarbonate–carbonic acid system is the most important plasma buffer system. We will use it as our baseline measure of changes in acid-base balance. Substitution of the values of sodium bicarbonate concentration and carbonic acid in the equation is done indirectly. It is difficult to measure the carbonic acid concentration in the plasma. We can estimate its value, however, by measuring the Pco$_2$ by a gas electrode and multiplying this figure by 0.03, which is the solubility constant of CO$_2$. The result is the equivalent of the carbonic acid concentration and has a value of approximately 1.2 mmole/liter, since the usual Pco$_2$ is 40 mm Hg. The bicarbonate can be measured directly or can be estimated by determining the total CO$_2$ content of the blood (25.2 mmole/liter) and then subtracting the CO$_2$ carried as carbonic acid (1.2 mmole/liter). The normal plasma value is thus 24 mmole/liter of bicarbonate. The pK of the carbonic acid system is 6.1; the normal blood pH is 7.4; and the normal ratio of bicarbonate to carbonic acid is 24:1.2, or more conveniently 20:1. A graph of the pH on the abscissa and the bicarbonate concentration on the ordinate yields a classic working diagram for studying acid-base imbalance (the *Davenport diagram*, presented in Fig. 5-7). The point (X) represented by a pH of 7.4, a Pco$_2$ of 40 mm Hg, and a bicarbonate concentration of 24 indicates the normal acid-base balance. Deviations from this point are also indicated. Each of these points will now be discussed separately. Continue to refer to the Davenport diagram as the various alterations are discussed. Table 5-5 summarizes the changes that occur in acid-base disorders.

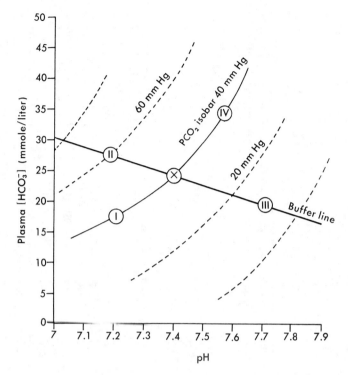

Fig. 5-7. Davenport diagram: classic working diagram for studying acid-base imbalance.

Any decrease in pH from 7.4 is the result of an incre se in free H^+ and is a state of acidosis. There are two major types of a idosis, metabolic (point I) and respiratory (point II). Notice that both are to the left of the normal pH of 7.4. The difference between these two states is therefore not of pH but of bicarbonate concentrations and Pco_2 values. In respiratory acidosis there is an increase in the Pco_2 and HCO_3^- concentration, and in metabolic acidosis a drop in bicarbonate concentration from the normal value of 24 mmole/liter occurs without a change in Pco_2. To understand this phenomenon, we need to once again examine the equation:

$$H_2O + CO_2 \rightleftarrows H_2CO_3 \rightleftarrows H^+ + HCO_3^-$$

When an increase in CO_2 occurs, it is apparent that through the law of mass action there will be a resultant increase in concentrations of both H^+ and HCO_3^-. Thus *respiratory acidosis*, which is characterized by both of these changes, is the result of a primary increase in Pco_2, which causes a rise in carbonic acid formation. Imagine a patient with severe pulmo-

Table 5-5. Alterations in the pH of body fluid*

Condition	Other names	Signs and symptoms	Sources	Compensatory mechanisms
Primary base bicarbonate deficit Ketones, chlorides, and/or organic acids replace $HCO_3^- \rightarrow$ deficit of base bicarbonate; ratio of 1 part H_2CO_3 to 20 parts HCO_3 is ↓ on HCO_3 side	Metabolic acidosis Primary alkali deficit Uncompensated alkali deficit Nonrespiratory acidosis	Deep, rapid breathing (Kussmaul) SOB on exertion Weakness Stupor Coma Laboratory findings Plasma pH ↓ 7.35 Urine pH ↓ 6 Plasma HCO_3 ↓ 25 mEq/ liter in adults and 20 mEq/ liter in children	Gain of strong acid by extracellular fluid Gain of exogenous acid Metabolic and organic acid overproduction and retention Loss of base from ECF Renal loss Intestinal loss	Respiratory: ↓ pH stimulates pulmonary ventilation; lungs blow off CO_2, and CO_2 is available to form H_2CO_3; acid side is decreased Renal: kidneys retain base bicarbonate through preferential excretion of $H^+ \rightarrow$ acid urine
Primary base bicarbonate excess Ratio of 1 part H_2CO_3 to 20 parts HCO_3 is ↑ on HCO_3 side, resulting in excess of base bicarbonate	Metabolic alkalosis Primary alkali excess Uncompensated alkali excess Nonrespiratory alkalosis	Depressed breathing (rate and depth) Hyperactive reflexes Muscle hypertonicity Tetany progressing to convulsions Laboratory findings Plasma pH ↑ 7.45 Urine pH ↑ 7.0 Plasma HCO_3 ↑ 25 mEq/ liter in adults and ↑ 20 mEq/liter in children Plasma K ↓ 4 mEq/liter	Gain of HCO_3 from ECF Gain of exogenous base Oxidation of salts of organic acids Loss of acid from ECF Intestinal loss Renal loss Potassium depletion (may be renal or extrarenal)	Respiratory: lungs hold back CO_2 to build up H_2CO_3 side; breathing may be shallow and irregular; ↑ Pco_2 of blood stimulates respiratory center Renal: kidneys excrete HCO_3 ions and retain H^+ and nonbicarbonate anions to aid in restoring ratio and pH to normal range → alkaline urine

Carbonic acid deficit of ECF Plasma Pco_2 ↓ because of hyperactive breathing; ratio of 1 part H_2CO_3 to 20 parts HCO_3 decreased on H_2CO_3 side	Respiratory alkalosis Hyperventilation Primary carbonic acid deficit Uncompensated carbonic acid deficit Hypocapnia Nonmetabolic alkalosis	Convulsions Tetany Unconsciousness Laboratory findings pH of plasma ↑7.45 pH of urine ↑7.0 Plasma HCO_3 ↓25 mEq/liter in adults and ↓20 mEq/liter in children	Anxiety, extreme emotion, hysteria Intentional overbreathing Rapid breathing (hyperpnea) Mechanical overventilation Oxygen lack High fever Encephalitis† Salicylate poisoning†	Renal: kidneys excrete HCO_3^- and retain H^+ and nonbicarbonate anions; urine becomes alkaline; by dropping bicarbonate level proper ratio is nearly restored
Carbonic acid excess of ECF Retention of CO_2 by the lungs causes an excess of carbonic acid; ratio of 1 part H_2CO_3 to 20 parts HCO_3 increased on H_2CO_3 side	Respiratory acidosis Primary CO_2 excess Uncompensated CO_2 excess Nonmetabolic acidosis Hypoventilation Hypercapnia	Respiratory embarrassment Weakness Coma Disorientation Laboratory findings Plasma pH ↓6.0 Urine pH ↓6.0 Plasma HCO_3 ↑29 mEq/liter in adults and ↑25 mEq/liter in children	Any condition that causes retention of carbon dioxide Asthma Chronic obstructive lung disease (COLD) Pneumonia Occlusion of breathing passages Barbiturate or morphine poisoning (causes depression of respiratory center)	Renal: kidneys conserve base bicarbonate while excreting H^+ and nonbicarbonate anions → acid urine

*From Groër, M. E., and Shekleton, M. E.: Basic pathophysiology: a conceptual approach, St. Louis, 1979, The C. V. Mosby Co.
†Respiratory center directly affected.

nary edema, in which fluid prevents adequate alveolar ventilation. The CO_2 produced by metabolism thus does not exchange across the alveolar wall but rises in concentration in the body fluids. The patient's total CO_2 would increase, all changes easily seen by examining the equation on p. 115.

Now imagine a patient with a primary metabolic problem, such as uncontrolled diabetes mellitus. This patient would have a high concentration of ketone bodies in the blood. These acids require buffering by the blood buffers (discussed earlier). Therefore, as these acids diffuse from the liver, where they are formed from fat metabolism, they react with bicarbonate. Thus a drop in pH may not occur at first, but eventually the bicarbonate reserves, representing 50% of the total buffer base, become depleted, and the acids are not adequately buffered. The pH begins to drop, and a state of acidosis, accompanied by a fall in bicarbonate, ensues. This classic metabolic acidosis is represented by point I in Fig. 5-7.

Another important consideration must now be discussed as the Davenport diagram is examined. Notice the Pco_2 isobars that cross the buffer line. In the case of metabolic acidosis the Pco_2 does not change, since point I is on the normal Pco_2 isobar, which represents a Pco_2 of 40 mm Hg. The reason is that Pco_2 is the major regulator of respiration under normal circumstances. As the metabolic acids accumulate, they do form CO_2 according to the law of mass action, as illustrated previously. However, CO_2 is quickly removed from the plasma through the respiratory system, and thus no rise in Pco_2 occurs in pure uncompensated metabolic acidosis.

Alkalosis is the result of a drop in free H^+ and therefore of a rise in plasma pH. Again, there are two types, respiratory and metabolic (represented on the Davenport diagram by points III and IV). The condition of respiratory alkalosis is associated with a rise in pH above 7.4 and a drop in bicarbonate and Pco_2 values. This condition is associated with an increased excretion of CO_2. The most common clinical example of respiratory alkalosis is that of hyperventilation. The patient breathes rapidly and deeply and "blows off" excessive amounts of CO_2. This drops the plasma Pco_2. Turning once again to the equation on p. 115, we see that the law of mass action dictates that with a drop in CO_2 the reaction will shift to the left, toward the formation of CO_2, which of course will decrease the concentrations of both H^+ and HCO_3^-.

Metabolic alkalosis (point IV) is associated with a rise in pH, but in this case the HCO_3^- concentration is much higher than normal, and the P_{CO_2} is normal. This condition is caused by either a primary rise in blood bicarbonate or a primary drop in blood pH. Whichever condition occurs first, the other will follow according to the law of mass action. If there is some pathophysiologic alteration that results in a rise in the HCO_3^-, the equation will shift to the left, resulting in a decrease in free H^+ and an increased formation of H_2CO_3. As this is formed it is rapidly blown off as CO_2, so that no rise in P_{CO_2} occurs.

A useful generalization may be made from observing the points on the Davenport diagram (Fig. 5-7). Acid-base disorders that are primarily the result of respiratory problems cause shifts in pH that move up or down the buffer line. Shifts in pH caused by metabolic problems result in changes along the P_{CO_2} isobar. Furthermore, when the body compensates for acid-base alterations, it does so through either respiratory or renal mechanisms, as previously described. When compensation, usually for a metabolic problem, is respiratory, the direction of compensation will be up or down the buffer line, or for renal compensation, usually in the case of respiratory changes, the compensation will move up or down the P_{CO_2} isobar. The second Davenport diagram (Fig. 5-8) shows the directions of compensation for respiratory acidosis and alkalosis and for metabolic acidosis and alkalosis. In the case of respiratory acidosis the major mechanism of compensation is through renal excretion of H^+ and reabsorption of bicarbonate to buffer the increased H^+. Therefore a rise in the plasma pH and in the concentration of HCO_3^- will follow the renal mechanisms. However, since P_{CO_2} will be unaffected by these renal mechanisms, the point of compensation will move up the specific P_{CO_2} isobar that the uncompensated point represents. In most cases of respiratory acidosis the respiratory tract is unable to respond to the increased P_{CO_2}, since there is usually some pathology in this system causing the state of acidosis. Therefore the compensation for acidosis must come from the kidneys.

Respiratory mechanisms are often able to compensate for metabolic acidosis. The kidneys also may compensate, although their effects generally take much longer than the very fast respiratory response to lowered pH and increasing P_{CO_2}. If the primary response to metabolic acidosis is through respiratory hyperpnea, which will blow off CO_2 and thus maintain the P_{CO_2}, then the point of compensation will occur along the buffer line drawn from the initial point II. Thus the P_{CO_2} will decrease, and the concentration of H^+ will also fall according to the law of mass action. A point should be made here about compensation efficiency. Respiratory efficiency is less than renal efficiency in the sense that renal com-

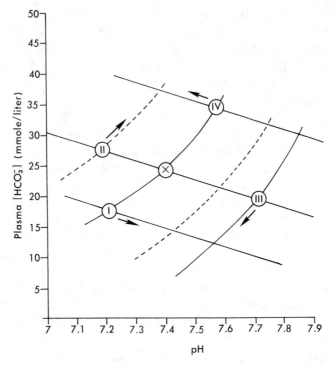

Fig. 5-8. Davenport diagram showing compensation for acidosis and alkalosis.

pensation can result in a return of the pH to the normal value of 7.4, whereas respiratory compensation usually cannot. It should also be recalled that the whole aim of compensation is a return of the body fluids to the normal pH, since it is the pH changes that are most dangerous to the body function—not the P_{CO_2} or the concentration of HCO_3^-. There is a very critical limit to pH changes that are compatible with survival (6.8 to 7.9) for any length of time; therefore compensation must restore the pH to as nearly normal as possible, as rapidly as possible.

Metabolic and respiratory alkalosis compensation follows the same general patterns as the compensation for the types of acidosis. Renal compensation occurs for respiratory alkalosis, and respiratory compensation occurs for metabolic alkalosis. Certainly there are many patients whose blood concentrations of bicarbonate and P_{CO_2} values reflect mixed compensation. However, for the purposes of clarity these points have been omitted from the graph (Fig. 5-7). Table 5-5 summarizes the biologic and clinical aspects of the four major acid-base disorders.

Respiratory acidosis

Etiology. Any condition that depresses respiration, mechanically impairs breathing, or impedes the diffusion of gases across the alveolar membrane can result in respiratory acidosis (also known as hypercapnia). Of course, the most dramatic example of acute respiratory acidosis is sudden respiratory arrest. In this case there is actually a combination of metabolic and respiratory acidosis, and large amounts of sodium bicarbonate must be given to the patient to buffer the excessive amounts of free H^+ that appear in the ECF. Gradations of respiratory failure also can occur. Patients with central nervous system (CNS) depression may have concurrent depression of the respiratory centers, which results in apneic spells, Cheyne-Stokes respiration, and other abnormal and inadequate respiratory patterns. Conditions that depress CNS respiratory control include profound sedation as the result of drug ingestion, traumatic head injuries, tumors, infectious processes such as meningitis, and cerebrovascular accidents. Mechanical ventilatory assistance is often required for the prevention of severe respiratory acidosis.

Other alterations in respiration leading to respiratory acidosis may be due to mechanical impairments of respiratory excursion. For example, traumatic injuries to the chest wall, poor expansion of the chest because of pain in the chest, back, or even abdomen, extreme obesity (Pickwickian syndrome), and certain neuromuscular diseases affecting the diaphragm or intercostal muscles may lead to inadequate ventilation at the alveolar level. Another cause of respiratory acidosis is obstruction of the air passages, such as the larnyx, bronchi, or bronchioles, which impedes air passage and also tremendously increases the work of breathing. Further causes include any conditions affecting the integrity of the alveolar membrane, such as emphysema, or interrupting the normal diffusional pathways for CO_2 and O_2 movement, such as pneumonia, cystic fibrosis, pulmonary edema, drowning, and pulmonary embolism.

It is important to realize that there are many patients with compensated respiratory acidosis. All patients surviving with serious chronic obstructive pulmonary disease (COPD) are not severely acidotic, since renal and, to some degree, respiratory compensation has allowed them to maintain a pH of close to 7.4. Such patients generally survive with very high P_{CO_2} levels, although there are many that actually have a peculiar pattern of blood gases; that is, they are extremely hyperpneic and through this compensation actually have a lowered P_{CO_2} and appear to be alkalotic! Generally, however, the patient with COPD has adapted to a high P_{CO_2}, has compensated by renal reabsorption of bicarbonate and excretion of

H^+, and has a nearly normal pH and a very high plasma concentration of bicarbonate. Such a chronic adaptation to high Pco_2 is in sharp contrast to the results of an abrupt change in Pco_2 from normal to high levels in a previously well individual. In the latter case the altered Pco_2 and resultant acidosis may be lethal.

Signs and symptoms. There is no clearly recognizable syndrome associated with respiratory acidosis. Most patients with a plasma pH of less than 7.2 have some signs of cerebral sedation, which may progress to coma. Some patients may have signs and symptoms associated with cerebral vasodilation and increased intracranial pressure caused by hypercapnia. These include a pounding occipital headache, dizziness, and confusion. If the hypercapnia results in hyperkalemia caused by cellular buffering, there may be signs and symptoms of potassium excess (Chapter 8). An eventual state of hypokalemia may result when the acidosis is corrected or in long-term states of hypercapnia. It is also important to remember that since disorders causing hypercapnia also usually interfere with oxygenation, hypoxia may be as life threatening as the hypercapnia.

Respiratory alkalosis

Etiology. The cause of respiratory alkalosis (hypocapnia) is increased ventilation resulting in excessive exhalation of CO_2. A variety of disorders may be responsible for this type of ventilatory pattern. The CNS control of respiratory rate and depth may be interrupted by drugs, infection, or tumors. The major drug class that, in excess, can directly stimulate the respiratory center is the salicylates. Thus aspirin overdosage does not immediately lead to metabolic acidosis, as one might expect, since aspirin is acidic. Rather, respiratory alkalosis results at first because of hyperventilation. A patient who is using a ventilator may be mechanically hyperventilated and may experience resultant hypocapnia. In such a patient the continual assessment of arterial blood gases and the clinical state is required. The most common cause of hyperventilation is anxiety. Persons who hyperventilate in response to fear, anxiety, or excitement usually have no awareness of their respiratory pattern and may come to the emergency room of the hospital after having "fainted" or become dizzy and lightheaded. Commonly these patients also complain of a feeling of breathlessness and tingling of the extremities, the latter probably the result of hypocalcemia caused by the effects of the higher pH on the free and bound calcium equilibrium (p. 181). Another cause of respiratory alkalosis is compensation for hypoxia or metabolic acidosis, in which the individual increases respiration to reduce Pco_2 and H^+. Other conditions occasionally associated with hypocapnia are fever, anemia, thyroid crisis, hypermetabolic states, exercise, and thiamine deficiency.

Like hypercapnia, hypocapnia may be a chronic condition associated with lowered Pco_2 and normal pH as the result of renal compensation. Persons who experience hypocapnia as a result of a chronic condition such as congestive heart failure or congenital heart disease are able to tolerate low levels of CO_2 that normally would be pathologic. When Pco_2 drops quickly, most individuals will suffer a variety of signs and symptoms. In making a diagnosis, one must recognize that respiratory alkalosis may be the result of some primary process or may be due to compensation for metabolic acidosis. Therefore the arterial blood gases, the pH, and the bicarbonate concentrations must be evaluated in conjunction with the patient's clinical picture.

A drop in Pco_2 will result in a drop in HCO_3^-, according to the law of mass action. The pH will rise only when the buffering capacity of the ECF is exceeded. The drop in bicarbonate is not great, as seen in the Davenport diagram (Fig. 5-7). The use of blood buffers such as hemoglobin and cellular buffering results in a release of H^+ into the ECF in the body's effort to maintain the proper pH. H^+ also must be made available to combine with HCO_3^- so that CO_2 is formed as quickly as the respiratory tract blows it off in respiratory alkalosis. Therefore other buffers contribute H^+, an phenomenon that helps to conserve the bicarbonate so that it does not fall greatly in the uncompensated state of respiratory alkalosis.

Signs and symptoms. As in respiratory acidosis, there is no one set of signs and symptoms that all patients will demonstrate. Many patients suffering acute hypocapnia will relate various paresthesias, such as tingling of the fingertips, numbness of the tongue, and generalized weakness. There may even be signs of tetany, such as carpopedal spasm and a positive Chvostek's sign. Convulsions may occur, or the patient may complain of faintness or dizziness. The anxious patient with the hyperventilation syndrome, usually a young female, may not be hyperventilating by the time she is seen by the nurse or physician. However, the signs and symptoms she describes may be mimicked by having her hyperventilate in the office. This is commonly done during chest auscultation by having the patient take repeated deep breaths as the examiner moves the stethoscope over the anterior, lateral, and posterior chest, pretending to listen to the breath sounds. Care must be taken, however, that the patient does not become excessively dizzy or faint, and consequently fall.

After this procedure the patient will often volunteer that the episode that brought her to seek health care was exactly the same as the experience of hyperventilation in the office. Restoration of the normal Pco_2 after acute hyperventilation can usually be achieved by having the patient rebreathe the expired air by breathing into a paper bag for a short time until the symptoms subside. Most patients with the hyperventilation syndrome, once they recognize the relationship of their ventilatory pattern with anxiety, are able to prevent further hyperventilation episodes.

Metabolic acidosis

Etiology. Metabolic acidosis results from a rise in H^+ concentration of the ECF caused either by a primary increase in H^+ or a decrease in bicarbonate and other buffer bases. Conditions that cause H^+ excess beyond the buffer capacity of the ECF include shock, dehydration, diabetic ketoacidosis or lactic acidosis, renal failure, ingestion of certain drugs (e.g., methanol), diarrhea, gastrointestinal tract fistulas, and renal tubular acidosis.

The two categories of metabolic acidosis, normochloremic and hyperchloremic, are classified according to the chloride concentration of the ECF. Whenever excess acids are introduced into the ECF, no matter what the cause, the effect on the HCO_3^- concentration is an inevitable drop, since HCO_3^- combines with H^+ to buffer H^+. Therefore metabolic acidosis is accompanied by a decrease in HCO_3^- concentration, as indicated on the Davenport diagram (Fig. 5-7). When bicarbonate drops, electrical neutrality must be maintained; thus the cations normally associated with it must be balanced by anions such as chloride. Thus, if the acid added to the ECF has Cl^- associated with it, then these anions will balance the cations, and electrical neutrality will be maintained. On the other hand, if the acidosis is due to the addition of acids without associated Cl^-, then there will be an increased "anion gap." The latter term is used to designate the sum of anions other than chloride and bicarbonate present in the ECF. Its normal value is approximately 16 mEq/liter. Conditions associated with a widened anion gap include salicylate poisoning, diabetic ketoacidosis, and lactic acidosis. Lactic acidosis is seen in hypoxia, in which the wastes of metabolism accumulate, aerobic metabolism halts, and large amounts of lactic acid accumulate in the tissues and the ECF. In this case the lactic acid is buffered by the sodium bicarbonate, resulting in formation of carbonic acid that is blown off by the lungs. The lactate anion then is retained to balance the cation according to the following reaction:

$$\text{Lactic acid} + \text{NaHCO}_3 \rightleftarrows \text{Na lactate} + \text{H}_2\text{CO}_3 \rightleftarrows \text{CO}_2 + \text{H}_2\text{O}$$

The lactate widens the anion gap, as predicted, since Cl^- is not associated with it.

Several different types of electrolyte problems can arise in the patient with metabolic acidosis. For example, the acid anions may be excreted through the kidneys while bicarbonate reabsorption continues. There may thus be a concomitant loss of Na^+ and K^+ in the urine to balance the acid anions. A further problem may be related to the cellular buffering, which causes Na^+ and K^+ to move out of the cells in exchange for H^+. Intracellular K^+ depletion results, and the ECF may be hyperkalemic. However, the excess K^+ is excreted by the kidney, and an eventual state of hypokalemia is possible. When the acidosis is treated, the K^+ will move back into the cells, and a profound state of hypokalemia can occur in response. The patient's cardiac function can be severely threatened by either the excess or deficit of potassium.

Signs and symptoms. Metabolic acidosis may first be recognized by the compensatory respiratory effort the patient makes. Thus, in diabetic acidosis, a characteristic pattern of breathing—Kussmaul's respirations—indicates that the patient is attempting to blow off excess CO_2 and thus maintain the pH level. Other signs and symptoms may be related to K^+ excess (Chapter 8). Weakness is usually present, and if acidosis is severe, there will be profound effects on CNS integrity, and coma will inevitably occur if acidosis is not compensated for nor treated. The compensation for metabolic acidosis is hyperpnea, as well as renal reabsorption of bicarbonate and excretion of H^+. The net effect is therefore to decrease the Pco_2, increase the pH, and restore bicarbonate. Note, however, that the Davenport diagram showing compensation effects (Fig. 5-8) indicates that the compensation for metabolic acidosis actually results in a fall in bicarbonate. Using the Henderson-Hasselbalch equation, calculate the ratio of bicarbonate to carbonic acid needed to maintain the pH at the compensated value of 7.32, as indicated on the diagram (Fig. 5-8):

$$\text{pH} = \text{pK} + \log \frac{\text{HCO}_3^-}{\text{H}_2\text{CO}_3}$$

$$7.32 = 6.1 + \log X$$
$$\log X = 7.32 - 6.1$$
$$\log X = 1.22$$
$$X = \text{antilog } 1.22$$
$$X = 16$$

The ratio of bicarbonate to carbonic acid should be 16:1. You can double-check this calculation by looking at the Davenport diagram and noting that the P_{CO_2} is about 32 mm Hg. Multiply this figure by 0.03 to obtain the value of H_2CO_3, and then divide the bicarbonate concentration at the point of compensation by this value. The number should closely correspond with the answer obtained through the use of the Henderson-Hasselbalch equation.

Metabolic alkalosis

Etiology. Metabolic alkalosis occurs as the result of a rise in the ECF concentration of HCO_3^- and a consequent increase in the plasma pH. The most common cause of this condition is protracted vomiting in which excessive acid is lost from the stomach. Normally the stomach contents are highly acid, with carbonic anhydrase present in the gastric luminal cells. This enzyme converts CO_2 to H^+, which is secreted into the stomach, and to HCO_3^-, which is reabsorbed. Excessive loss of stomach H^+, with accompanying Cl^-, will cause both a rise in ECF pH and hypochloremia. According to the law of mass action, the equation on p. 115 will be driven to the right, toward the formation of H^+ and HCO_3^-. As a result the bicarbonate concentration will rise, helping to balance the loss of Cl^- that usually occurs in vomiting. Metabolic alkalosis may result from any type of gastric drainage, such as through a nasogastric tube attached to suction.

Other causes of metabolic alkalosis include the milk-alkali syndrome. This condition is the result of the ingestion of large amounts of milk and drugs such as sodium bicarbonate by persons with gastric acidity disturbances. It can result in a sufficient change in blood pH to cause a state of alkalosis, especially in persons with decreased renal function. Certain drugs, including steroids and diuretics, can produce metabolic alkalosis. It may also develop in patients with hyperaldosteronism or Cushing's syndrome. The reason is that aldosterone and corticosteroids, in general, increase Na^+ reabsorption in the distal convoluted tubule (DCT). This mechanism results in Na^+ uptake coupled to K^+ or H^+ secretion into the tubular filtrate. Therefore, when excessive amounts of these hormones are present, Na^+ is retained and H^+ is lost; thus a state of alkalosis eventually develops.

When chloride concentration is decreased in the ECF, there is an increase in Na^+ and HCO_3^- reabsorption from the DCT, with resultant loss of H^+ and K^+ into the urine because of the linkage of Na^+ reabsorption to H^+ and K^+ secretion. The plasma concentration of HCO_3^- is maintained at a high level by this mechanism to provide an electrochemical balance to the body fluids. Interestingly, a person with chloride depletion and resultant metabolic alkalosis secretes an acid urine, since bicarbonate must be reabsorbed to balance the body cations, and this process results in Na^+ reabsorption and H^+ secretion. Obviously the treatment for such a patient is provision of chloride, which will then result in a loss of bicarbonate in the urine and a return to normal acid-base balance.

Metabolic alkalosis may be a confusing entity to diagnose unless the patient's history, physical examination, and blood gases and chemistries are carefully evaluated. The Davenport diagram (Fig. 5-7) should be closely examined so that the differences between metabolic alkalosis and chronic respiratory disorders with compensated respiratory acidosis are clear. The arterial Pco_2 in metabolic alkalosis is usually at or near normal, whereas the Pco_2 in chronic hypercapnia is much greater than normal.

Compensation for metabolic alkalosis is indicated in the Davenport diagram (Fig. 5-8). Here it is seen that the primary means of compensation is respiratory hypocapnia. The high pH inhibits the medullary respiratory centers and decreases the rate and depth of respirations, thus reducing the amount of Pco_2 blown off by the lungs, which in turn increases the Pco_2, increases carbonic acid, and increases both HCO_3^- and H^+ concentrations. Thus, in compensation, even more bicarbonate is added to the ECF, and the increased H^+ concentration drops the pH toward the normal range. The limitation of this compensation is arterial Po_2, since a drop in this value is a potent stimulant of the respiratory centers through the carotid and aortic chemoreceptors.

Signs and symptoms. Metabolic alkalosis is usually identified as the result of another disease entity. It may be diagnosed when a patient has been vomiting for several days or after prolonged diuretic therapy. It is frequently seen along with hypokalemia, since in this state there is an exchange of H^+ for K^+ both at the cellular level and at the level of the tubule. Since K^+ is saved and H^+ is lost, a drop in H^+ and metabolic alkalosis results. Signs and symptoms associated with decreases in chloride or potassium are described in other chapters of this book. No particular set of signs and symptoms associated with metabolic alkalosis is readily identifiable. Even the respiratory depression, which is the major compensatory mechanism, is difficult to assess when the metabolic alkalosis is mild.

Case study: a premature infant with metabolic acidosis

The case study on pp. 129 to 131 demonstrates several aspects of acid-base balance. Depending on the client and the derangement, there may be no easily recognizable, observable signs and symptoms. Taking a good history and frequently monitoring the blood gases and blood chemistries are essential. The nurse's assessment of the patient is important, since small changes may have great relevance to a changing acid-base balance. Thus, in this tiny patient, the only clues to a changing acid-base state were history, altered feeding, and weight loss.

The case study presented below illustrates the interesting condition of late metabolic acidosis (LMA), which occurs most frequently in premature infants. Its occurrence is related to two major factors: the inability of the kidneys to handle an acid load and the type of formula the infant receives. The metabolism of protein results in the production of acids, which are excreted through urinary acidification and buffered by HCO_3^- reabsorption. When the immature renal tubules are presented with a high acid load, there is a possibility of metabolic acidosis. Furthermore, when renal hypoxia occurs as the result of birth stress and hypoxia in the premature infant, renal tubules are damaged and the renal function is even further depressed. Infant formulas contain variable degrees of protein, as can be seen in Table 5-6. The actual protein needs of the premature infant are unknown, but it is clear that protein metabolism results in an increased acid load on the kidneys, which can lead to late metabolic acidosis as seen in the infant described in the case study. There is a greater likelihood of LMA in infants fed formula high in casein as contrasted to those fed whey-predominant formula (such as human milk). The symp-

Table 5-6. Caloric and protein concentration of commonly used formulas*

Formulas	Caloric concentration (kcal/oz)	Protein (gm/ 100 ml)	Protein (gm/ 100 kcal)	Percentage of kcal as protein	Whey- casein ratio
Human milk	—	1.1	1.5	7	60:40
Similac	20	1.5	2.3	9.3	18:82
	24	2.2	2.7	11	18:82
Enfamil	20	1.5	2.3	9	18:82
	24	1.8	2.3	9	18:82
Isomil	20	2.0	3.0	12	
	24	2.4	3.0	12	
SMA	20	1.5	2.2	9	60:40
	24	1.8	2.3	9	
Portagen	20	2.3	3.3	9	0:100
PM 60/40	20	1.6	2.4	13.6	60:40
Nutramigen	20	2.2	3.3	13	0:100
Enfamil Premature	24	2.2	2.8	11	18:82

*From Brockemyre, P., and Schreiner, R. L.: J. Am. Diet. Assoc. **72:**298, 1978. Copyright The American Dietetic Association. Reprinted with permission from the Journal of The American Dietetic Association.

toms exhibited by the infant are vague in comparison with those of the adult with metabolic acidosis. For example, the hyperpnea expected as a sequela of respiratory compensation was only very slight in the infant discussed in the case study. Nevertheless, respiratory compensation occurred because the Pco_2 decreased. The major symptoms of this form of metabolic acidosis is failure to gain weight (or loss of weight). There may be anorexia, lethargy, and increased respiratory rate, but these symptoms may also be absent. The treatment is restoration of blood base by administration of bicarbonate or feeding of nonnitrogenous formula, such as glucose water, until the blood values return to normal and the infant begins to gain weight. In premature infants who have suffered renal hypoxia, there is an amazing recovery of kidney function as compared to the adult, and even without treatment most cases of late metabolic acidosis resolve without incident.

CASE STUDY • LATE METABOLIC ACIDOSIS IN A PREMATURE INFANT

IDENTIFYING DATA
Baby Boy J., a 9-day-old white infant in the intensive care nursery (ICN), developed metabolic acidosis.

FAMILY HISTORY
The baby's mother was 22 years old, and her one previous pregnancy had resulted in a stillbirth. Baby J. was delivered by cesarean section at 30 weeks' gestation because of placenta previa and premature onset of labor.

HISTORY
The baby's Apgar scores 1 and 5 minutes after delivery were 5 and 7, respectively. Resuscitation by bag and mask was required in the delivery room, and the infant was immediately transferred to the ICN. All premature infants are at risk for the development of metabolic acidosis; however, Baby J. was at increased risk because he experienced many stresses during the first few days of life that may have caused a degree of renal asphyxia. When the infant was admitted to the nursery, the physical examination revealed mild intercostal retractions with grunting respirations, bilaterally decreased breath sounds, poor muscle tone, and absent Moro and suck reflexes. The rest of the physical examination was within normal limits. The initial vital signs and laboratory values were as follows:

Vital signs	*Laboratory values*	
Temperature: 35.7° C (96.2°F)	Bilirubin: 2.0 mg/dl	pH: 7.104
Heart rate: 146	Glucose: 50 mg/dl	Pco_2: 62.9 mm Hg
Respirations: 50	Hematocrit: 54.4%	Pao_2: 20.0 mm Hg
Weight: 1410 gm	Hemoglobin: 19 gm/dl	HCO_3: 19.7 mEq

The initial chest x-ray film revealed hyperexpanded lungs and fluid in the major lung fissures, suggesting a diagnosis of respiratory distress syndrome, type 2. The baby was intubated with an endotracheal tube and placed on a respirator with intermittent mandatory ventilation and positive end expiratory pressure and with a forced inspiratory oxygen (FIO$_2$) of 100%.

Shortly after admission to the ICN, Baby J. began to show signs of increasing respiratory distress, and a tentative diagnosis of persistent fetal circulation was made. After treatment with a tolazoline (Priscoline) infusion (1 mg/ml at 2 ml/hr), the baby's respiratory status gradually improved. Blood gas analyses were done frequently during the first four days, and the ranges of values were as follows:

pH: 7.14 to 7.409
Pco$_2$: 27 to 50.9 mm Hg
Pao$_2$: 25.7 to 137 mm Hg
HCO$_3$: 15.2 to 23.5 mEq

A diminished urinary output was noted during the first 2 days of the infant's life and was attributed to possible renal asphyxia leading to failure.

On the second day of life the baby was placed on continuous positive airway pressure in room air. The endotracheal tube was removed on the third day, and the baby was placed in an oxygen hood with an FIO$_2$ of 36%. On the fourth day of life Baby J. no longer required ventilatory assistance and was placed in room air. The blood gas values at this time were as follows:

pH: 7.347
Pco$_2$: 33.9 mm Hg
Pao$_2$: 81.3 mm Hg
HCO$_3$: 18.2 mEq

No further blood gas studies were done until the baby was 9 days old.

HISTORY OF PRESENT ILLNESS

Nasogastric feedings of Similac 20 were initiated gradually on the fourth day of life when the infant began to diurese. The following list of the infant's weights over the first 9 days of life demonstrates an initial weight gain over the first 3 days caused by fluid retention resulting from renal failure. The diuresis typical of recovery from renal failure, which occurred on the fourth day, resulted in a considerable weight loss (174 gm). The slow pattern of weight gain between the fourth and eighth days and the loss of 30 gm between the eighth and ninth days suggested a problem with *metabolic acidosis*. The baby's weights were as follows:

Age (days)	Weight (gm)
1	1410
2	1430
3	1450
4	1276
5	1262
6	1247

Age (days)	Weight (gm)
7	1300
8	1300
9	1270

The following blood gas values were obtained on the ninth day, and the diagnosis of late metabolic acidosis was confirmed.

pH: 7.30
Pco_2: 29.3 mm Hg
Pao_2: 72.8 mm Hg
HCO_3: 14.5 mEq

The baby was treated with a solution of sodium bicarbonate (2 mEq) added to each of two successive feedings. The treatment was considered successful because of the subsequent improvement in the baby's pattern of weight gain, and no further blood gas analyses were done. The infant's weights on the 4 days after treatment were as follows:

Age (days)	Weight (gm)
10	1300
11	1320
12	1360
13	1380

NURSING IMPLICATIONS AND DISCHARGE PLANNING

Prevention of unnecessary stress on premature infants requires that laboratory procedures be performed only when considered essential; blood gas analyses are not done routinely after the infant's respiratory status has improved. All premature infants, and particularly those who have had problems with hypoxia or asphyxia, are at risk for the development of metabolic acidosis during the first few weeks of life. Nurses need to carefully evaluate the early growth patterns of such infants because poor weight gain is the primary symptom of LMA. Prior to Baby J.'s hospital discharge, his parents should be provided with information about expected patterns of infant weight gain and should be advised to have the baby's weight checked periodically on a reliable scale. The use of high-protein formulas may predispose premature infants to the development of metabolic acidosis because the infant's immature kidneys are unable to handle the quantity of acid released by protein catabolism. Breast-fed premature infants rarely develop late metabolic acidosis. Another discharge planning consideration for this family, therefore, is the need for Mr. and Ms. J. to understand their baby's nutritional requirements. A blood gas analysis should be repeated if the infant shows any further signs of metabolic acidosis.

6

Volume disturbances

This chapter will describe the two major kinds of volume disturbances, volume deficit (dehydration) and volume excess (overhydration). Both conditions involve alterations in the total body water, affecting either the ECF or the ICF. Dehydration and overhydration are not disease entities in themselves but, rather, are signs of underlying disorders. However, these volume disorders can be life threatening and occasionally require emergency treatment, even before the underlying pathology can be identified and treated. Many compensatory mechanisms operate to maintain the steady state in the face of volume disorders, and medical and nursing approaches are often directed at supporting those coping mechanisms that ensure survival, as well as attempting to correct the condition itself. This chapter will describe the common volume disorders, the causes of each condition, the physiologic compensatory mechanisms that come into play, and nursing assessment and strategies aimed at early detection of serious pathophysiology. Treatment of each condition will also be summarized, and a case study will exemplify the clinical presentation of dehydration.

DEHYDRATION

The term *dehydration* describes a state of water deficit that is beyond the normal regulatory systems of the body to repair. In normal circumstances water output is balanced by intake through mechanisms described in detail in Chapter 2. If the water output is so excessive that intake cannot match it, the first effect is a state of ECF volume deficit. The guiding principle for determination of the effects on plasma osmolarity in all cases of fluid loss is first to look at the osmolarity of that fluid and then to examine the osmolarity of any fluids that have been ingested or infused in an attempt to repair the loss. Obviously, if no water is ingested or infused in an individual who has lost pure plasma or ECF, the ECF left behind will be of smaller volume, but its composition and osmolarity will not be affected. The various compensatory mechanisms of the body function to maintain cardiovascular function and perfusion of vital centers in volume losses. Other mechanisms act to conserve the body water or to actually repair the loss. Thus a major effect of dehydration is sympathetic nervous system activation, which will result in vasoconstriction of the arterioles, conservation of blood pressure, and perfusion of the heart, lungs, and brain. Vasodilation of vessels supplying the skeletal muscles also occurs, with the result that increased blood supply occurs there. Another effect of volume deficit is a drop in renal blood flow (RBF) and glomerular filtration rate (GFR), with the result that urine output is decreased, ensuring that water will be retained in the ECF rather than excreted. In fact, one of the earliest signs of dehydration is a drop in urine volume from its normal value of 1 ml/min (50 to 60 ml/hr). Thirst may also be stimulated through the hypertonic swelling and shrinking mechanisms of the thirst centers in the hypothalamus, as described in Chapter 2, in cases of hypertonic dehydration. When isotonic fluid loss has occurred, volume receptors supply information to the hypothalamus, stimulating the thirst centers and also the hypothalamic nuclei involved in the secretion of ADH. Volume receptors are believed to be present in the right atrium and vena cava, with sensory nerve fibers traveling to the hypothalamus. Aldosterone secretion is also stimulated, causing renal reabsorption of Na^+ and water to increase.

Since most states of dehydration involve loss of solute and water in proportion to the amounts contained within the ECF, the serum osmolarity is unaffected in the primary untreated condition. However, if a person suffering from dehydration replaces the fluid loss with either plain water or very hypertonic fluid containing a high concentration of electrolytes, there will be resultant alterations in the ECF and ICF. Imagine replacement of isotonic fluid loss with plain water. The water ingested will dilute both the ECF and sodium, which is the major cation of the ECF. A state of ECF hyponatremia then results. The lowered osmotic pressure of the ECF causes net movement of water into the cells, producing ECF dehydration and ICF overhydration. Of course, the ECF hyponatremia may result in symptoms associated with sodium deficit (Chapter 7), or the major symptoms may be related to the ECF dehydration. On the other hand, ingestion of a salty solution in cases of isotonic water loss causes a reversal of the above situation. The excessive sodium is trapped in the ECF and is osmotically active, resulting in a hypertonic

ECF and, because of osmosis out of cells, a dehydration of the cells. This condition, known as hypernatremic dehydration, results in agonizing thirst but few cardiovascular symptoms, since the ECF volume is normal or even sometimes increased.

Thus we can see that dehydration as a clinical entity has three forms: isotonic, hyponatremic (or hyposmolar), and hypernatremic (or hyperosmolar) dehydration. Each of these conditions and their causes and treatment will be discussed separately. It is crucial that nurses be able to recognize the differences between these forms of dehydration.

Isotonic dehydration

Etiology. Many situations can result in the loss of ECF, but the most common one is loss from the gastrointestinal tract such as might occur with vomiting, diarrhea, or drainage from fistulas or tubes. Gastrointestinal fluid is nearly isotonic with ECF. Another common pathologic condition, known as "third spacing," consists of isotonic fluid compartmentalization in a space such as the abdominal cavity, a joint, or other space from which fluid is not easily exchangeable with the ECF. Thus for all practical purposes this fluid, while still contained within the body, is nevertheless sequestered from the fluid exchange that is necessary for the maintenance of dynamic equilibrium. It is possible in some third-spacing syndromes for the fluid to be returned to the ECF when the underlying pathology is corrected, but in most cases removal of the fluid is accomplished through mechanical means, such as paracentesis. Loss of plasma or whole blood also represents isotonic fluid loss. Plasma loss such as occurs in burns may result in hemoconcentration, in that the hematocrit of the blood is increased because the volume of plasma in which the erythrocytes are contained is decreased. However, there is no important effect on the solutes contained within the plasma itself. It is important to note that although isotonic losses do not cause alterations in the concentrations of the various electrolytes dissolved in the ECF, there is usually, nevertheless, a drop in the total body amounts of these solutes. Thus, with correction of the volume deficit, there may be a concomitant decrease in the concentration of these solutes unless they are also replaced.

Another important cause of isotonic loss is excessive sensible perspiration. This is not a true isotonic loss, since sweat is slightly hypotonic. Thus there may be slightly more water than solute lost in excessive diaphoresis, leaving behind a very slightly hypertonic ECF. Most authorities consider this loss to be isotonic, however. It is important to recognize the differences between sensible and insensible perspiration through the skin. The latter is loss of water only, values for which were given in Chapter 2.

Excessive diaphoresis is often followed by excessive ingestion of large amounts of tap water, which results in dilution of the ECF, hyponatremia, and cellular dehydration. Many athletes now guard themselves against these problems by drinking electrolyte-containing "sports" fluids. These same liquids have become valuable adjuncts in the treatment of diarrhea and other conditions causing electrolyte deficiencies.

When a contraction of the ECF occurs, the major compensatory responses that can be assessed by the nurse are related to the activation of the sympathetic nervous system (SNS). Table 6-1 shows how the percentage of dehydration is related to fluid and weight loss and indicates the accompanying symptoms. Generally patients with a 3% or greater dehydration show signs and symptoms related to SNS activation.

The degree of activation of the SNS is dependent on the percentage of dehydration and the coping ability of the individual. Hypovolemic shock is the outcome of severe dehydration of the ECF and is characterized by widespread SNS activation as the major body defense reaction. The effects of hypovolemic shock, as in all forms of shock, are related to decreased cardiac output, decreased tissue perfusion, and eventual irreversible microcirculatory damage if treatment of hypovolemia is not carried out. This phenomenon can be understood by examining, at various levels, the effects of the widespread SNS activation that occurs with hypovolemia.

SNS response. The major activation of the vasogenic sympathetic centers located in the hypothalamus and medulla is through the stimulation of (1) nerves ending in the carotid and aortic sinuses and (2) atrial volume receptors. These nerve endings are sensitive to pressure and volume of the blood as it passes through the carotid artery, aortic arch, and atrium. Expansion of blood volume and pressure is the result of hypervolemia, and a drop in blood volume and pressure is related to hypovolemia. Fig. 6-1 diagrams the mechanism through which blood pressure is regulated

Table 6-1. Fluid and weight loss in dehydration

	Mild	Moderate	Severe
Infants	5% (50 ml/kg)	10% (100 ml/kg)	15% (150 ml/kg)
Adults	3% (30 ml/kg)	5% (60 ml/kg)	9% (90 ml/kg)

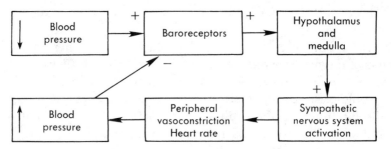

Fig. 6-1. Baroreceptors in carotid and aortic sinuses respond to fall in blood pressure by increasing sympathetic outflow. Pressure may be restored through cardiovascular effects of catecholamines.

by sympathetic outflow from the central nervous system. When blood volume or pressure increases, these baroreceptors are stimulated, resulting in a signal to the involved centers in the brain to decrease the rate of firing of the sympathetic nerves and, often, to increase parasympathetic outflow. Conversely, a drop in pressure or volume of the blood results in a variable decrease in the rate of firing of the baroreceptor nerves. This decrease inhibits parasympathetic nervous system activity and increases the sympathetic activation. Dehydration of 3% or more causes a sympathetic response through these mechanisms. The effects of the sympathetic activation are mainly cardiovascular, although other effects do occur. With regard to the heart, the catecholamines (epinephrine and norepinephrine) released during this hypovolemic stress cause the myocardium to exert greater contractile strength. The result is an increase in stroke volume, with less end systolic volume contained within the ventricles. The heart rate is also increased markedly through the effects of epinephrine and norepinephrine on the slope of the pacemaker potential. Since this slope is increased, more impulses are generated from the sinoatrial node in a given unit of time. The slope of the pacemaker potential, it will be recalled, is a measure of the speed of depolarization of the cells within the sinoatrial node. The catecholamines also increase the conduction speed of the pacemaker-generated impulses throughout the myocardium. The net result of these physiologic effects is a faster heart rate and an increase in the force of contraction of each beat of the heart. There is also a dangerous predisposition of the catecholamine-stimulated heart to arrhythmias, particularly ventricular extrasystoles (premature ventricular contractions) and ventricular fibrillation. This predisposition is due to an increased sensitivity of Purkinje's fibers, so that they are more likely to set up ectopic foci, which can stimulate the heart to contract inappropriately.

It is apparent that the beneficial cardiac effects assist the patient in maintaining the cardiac output even when the actual blood volume has been decreased through dehydration. Cardiac output (flow; $\dot{Q}$) is equal to heart rate multiplied by stroke volume:

$$\dot{Q} = HR \times SV$$

An increase in either the heart rate or the stroke volume causes an increase in the cardiac output, and perfusion of tissues will thus be maintained. The main danger early in hypovolemic shock is decreased oxygenation and nutrition of the vital centers that maintain life—the heart and brain. For perfusion to be adequate, the flow of blood going to the tissue through the arterioles must have sufficient pressure to overcome the resistance to flow that these vessels offer. Obviously, if these vessels are tightly constricted, the blood must be pushed through these high-resistance vessels with a considerable amount of pressure. When blood volume decreases, the hydrostatic pressure of the blood also naturally decreases.

Another effect of SNS activation is arteriolar constriction. Recall that the arterioles are the major resistance vessels of the cardiovascular tree. The greatest amount of pressure drop occurs along these vessels: blood enters the arterioles with a mean pressure of about 100 mm Hg and then leaves them and enters the capillaries with a pressure of approximately 32 mm Hg. These vessels offer such great resistance to blood flow because of their anatomic structure and physiologic regulation. The arterioles branch extensively off small arteries and are of small caliber. Smooth muscle is present within their linings and in the precapillary and postcapillary sphincters, and contraction of the smooth vessel results in constriction of the arteriole, causing a decreased diameter of the vessel. The smooth muscle is affected by several factors. Metabolites produced by the tissue that the arterioles supply can accumulate, and when a critical concentration is reached, there is a local vasodilation of the arterioles. The effect of this response is to open up the arterioles so that the blood flow through the capillary bed will increase. The result is (1) transport of the metabolites into the venous side of the circulation for eventual disposal through the lungs or liver and (2) increased oxygenation of the tissue so that metabolism will be stimulated. The metabolites are often reutilized in various pathways by the cells. The size of the arterioles is also regulated by the nervous system through sympathetic nerves, which release norepinephrine from their terminals. Parasympathetic nerves also supply parts of the cardiovascular tree. The effect of the neurotransmitters released by these nerves is to contract or relax the arteriolar smooth muscle walls and the smooth muscle of the precapillary and postcapillary sphincters, venules, and larger veins. The general effect of SNS stimulation is vasoconstriction, except in the skeletal muscle vessels, which respond by vasodilation. This difference in effect is due to the relative proportion of α-adrenergic and β-adrenergic receptors in different tissues. The response of α-adrenergic receptors to norepinephrine is vasoconstriction, and β-adrenergic receptor activation causes vasodilation. The result on blood pressure when there is widespread arteriolar constriction is obvious from the following formula, which is a modification of Ohm's law:

$$\dot{Q} = \frac{\Delta P}{R}$$

This formula states that the blood flow (or cardiac output) is proportional to the change in pressure that occurs as the blood is dynamically ejected from the left ventricle and opposed by the resistance to flow that the cardiovascular tree offers. By constricting arterioles, SNS activation increases the total peripheral resistance to blood flow ejected from the heart. If the above equation is restated, it can be seen that

$$P = \dot{Q} \times R$$

Thus pressure can be maintained, if flow decreases, only by an increase in resistance. Blood flow in hypovolemia is maintained centrally, to the heart and brain, at the expense of the peripheral vascular beds.

During hypovolemic stress, the SNS is activated and the level of blood catecholamines rises dramatically. Cardiac output is maintained through SNS activation as described, but widespread vasoconstriction in peripheral arterioles is an additional effect. As can be seen in the equation, vasoconstriction, by increasing resistance, will maintain blood pressure even when cardiac output falls, as always occurs in hypovolemic shock. Thus blood pressure is maintained in early shock, but cardiac output is decreased. If fluid continues to be lost from the ECF, the cardiac output continues to fall, but blood pressure can be maintained until 30% of the actual blood volume is decreased. Thereafter, blood pressure drops precipitously. When a hypovolemic patient has a significant drop in blood pressure, the patient is in shock and thus is in extreme danger of developing irreversible microcirculatory damage.

During the early responses to hypovolemia, the arteriolar vasocon-

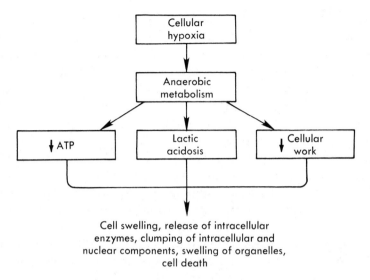

Fig. 6-2. Results of prolonged cellular hypoxia.

striction maintains blood pressure, but at the expense of certain tissues. Since less blood can flow through constricted arterioles offering high resistance, tissue perfusion is decreased, and hypoxia of the tissue results. The splanchnic organs (particularly the kidneys), skin, and muscle receive less perfusion than normal, and the blood is shunted to the heart and brain. The heart and brain are spared the effects of SNS-stimulated arteriolar constriction because the vessels supplying these organs lack a significant number of α-adrenergic receptors. The regulation of blood supply is through local autoregulation of vascular tone, and the shock state must be profound before the heart and brain suffer decreased flow. This regulation is, of course, a necessary aspect of the coping responses of the body to hypovolemia, since the heart and brain are the organs involved in the response to, and compensation of, this state. However, the peripheral tissue, underperfused and hypoxic, is naturally threatened by an extended period of vasoconstriction. Both the length and degree of peripheral vasoconstriction are important determinants of the degree of hypoxic damage that can result. Fig. 6-2 illustrates how cellular hypoxia damages the cells by interrupting the normal cell physiology. The switch to anaerobic metabolism that occurs during hypoxia causes an overall depression in the production of ATP. Therefore cellular contraction, transport, anabolism, secretion, and mitosis—processes requiring a source of metabolic energy—become disturbed and depressed. The cells accumulate sodium, lose potassium, and swell osmotically, losing their morphologic and physiologic integrity. Endothelial cells lining the blood vessels themselves are subject to hypoxic injury, as are cells throughout the tissues involved. Although the theory is controversial, many authorities believe that devastating hypoxic damage to capillary endothelium forms the basis of irreversibility in progressive shock.

Early in the SNS activation during hypovolemia, the effects of peripheral vasoconstriction are observable. One very early sign of dehydration is a decrease in urine volume. It is due in part to an increase in ADH and aldosterone, both released as soon as hypovolemic stress is detected by volume receptors and the juxtaglomerular apparatus. These hormones will cause net water and salt reabsorption in the tubules and collecting ducts of the kidneys. The major cause of oliguria is the renal vascular constriction, which causes a marked drop in RBF, GFR, and urine output. The normal autoregulatory mechanisms of the kidney are not effective in hypovolemic shock, in which SNS stimuli directly result in vasoconstriction of the renal arterioles. The drop in urine volume may not be particularly striking in early dehydration. The normal urine output in the adult male is 50 to 60 ml/hr, and this amount may be reduced only slightly with mild dehydration of 3% to 5%. However, as dehydration progresses to a moderate or marked stage, oliguria may be severe and is an important clinical sign. Accompanying the oliguria are signs of azotemia, since the kidneys are not able to excrete nitrogenous wastes adequately. A decrease in urinary output to 30 ml/hr or less in an adult is evidence of renal underperfusion. There is danger that the renal hypoxia will cause acute tubular necrosis and renal failure, even if the patient recovers from the hypovolemic episode. Therefore assessment of output is absolutely vital in dehydration, and an indwelling catheter should be placed in the bladder to monitor urine output. The specific gravity of the urine should also be carefully evaluated during the period of dehydration and during recovery.

Other signs of impending hypovolemic shock are also related to SNS-stimulated vasoconstriction. The skin is cold, pale or even cyanotic, occasionally mottled, and "clammy" to touch. The temperature and color are related to the decreased perfusion of the skin, and the moisture of the skin is related to SNS stimulation of the sweat glands. This relationship is paradoxic, since some fluid will be lost from an already dehydrated person through this response. However, the sweat glands do not receive dual innervation, and sympathetic stimulation causes sweating. The gastrointestinal tract and splanchnic organs are also underperfused and can become hypoxic in hypovolemic shock. It is believed that gut ischemia, induced by prolonged splanchnic vasoconstriction, contributes to the development of progressive irreversible shock. The gastrointestinal bacterial flora may be released into the systemic vasculature through ischemic, permeable intestinal mucosa. Since the liver's reticuloendothelial function is depressed because of hepatic hypoxia, sepsis results. The overwhelming sepsis may cause endotoxins and bacteria to ultimately destroy the normal permeability of the endothelium of capillaries throughout the cardiovascular tree, and even if the ECF is replaced, the vascular compartment cannot be maintained. This inability to maintain the vascular compartment is a characteristic of irreversible shock, in which no pharmacologic or fluid-and-electrolyte therapy can maintain the blood pressure and blood volume.

Since the cardiovascular system is most profoundly affected by SNS activity, the heart rate and the quality of the pulse are both measures of the efficacy of sympathetic stimulation. Early in hypovolemia, when dehydration is mild, the pulse rate is either normal or slightly increased, but the quality of the pulse is usually not altered. However, in moderate to severe dehydration, the pulse is not only rapid but thready in quality and in severe dehydration may be irregular as well. The blood pressure is maintained in mild dehydration through the SNS but begins to drop as hypovolemic shock develops. Systolic pressure values are between 60 and 90 mm Hg in moderate dehydration and in severe dehydration fall to extremely hypotensive levels.

Dehydration in infants, older children, and adults is classified according to the standard mild, moderate, and severe categories. The percentage of body weight lost (summarized in Table 6-1) differs for infants and for older children and adults.

A patient with mild dehydration may show few or mild symptoms other than weight loss, which cannot be ascertained unless an accurate weight measurement was obtained before the illness. Unfortunately, this measurement is rarely available. The loss of ECF may dry out the skin and mucous membranes, decreasing skin turgor. The patient may complain of thirst, but often this need may be elicited only during questioning and is not always a major drive. If dehydration progresses, the dryness of the mucous membranes becomes pronounced, and longitudinal furrows may be present on the tongue. Thirst is often severe. A sunken anterior fontanel and an absence of tears are noticeable in infants. Neck veins become flat, and small vein filling is decreased. Capillary filling is poor after blanching of the skin. The patient will usually exhibit some type of mental impairment, which may progress to actual coma in severe dehydration. The ability of a person to survive severe dehydration is dependent on age and general health, as well as on the severity of other problems such as metabolic acidosis and potassium imbalance. Since the presence of severe dehydration represents a state of hypovolemic shock that can rapidly become irreversible, recognition and prompt, appropriate treatment of the patient are paramount for survival.

Hypernatremic dehydration

Hypernatremic dehydration is a type of hypovolemia that is usually not characterized by the cardiovascular signs and ultimate circulatory collapse of isotonic dehydration. Rather, it results from loss of excess water from the ECF. The ECF becomes hyperosmolar, causing cellular dehydration with relative maintenance of the volume of the ECF. Hypernatremic dehydration (serum $Na^+ > 150$ mEq/liter) is usually associated with excessive insensible water loss (IWL). You will recall that the IWL is nearly pure water loss through the skin and lungs, and normally 20 to 40 ml/kg is lost each day through this route, the purpose of which is heat dissipation. Two thirds of the IWL is lost through the skin, and one third through evaporative lung losses. Metabolic increases, producing excess heat, will also increase IWL. For every milliliter of water lost through this route, approximately 0.58 calorie of heat is removed from the body. When fever is present, the excess heat load causes a rise in IWL of about 10% for every 1° C. Hyperventilation also increases IWL, as does a hot, dry environment. When IWL increases, the usual compensatory response of the body is an increase in water ingestion and a decrease in urinary water output. However, the thirst drive, which is so powerful in this type of dehydration, may not be apparent in the small infant, the elderly person, or any person with an altered mental status. Hypernatremia often develops quickly and is common in infantile diarrhea when lost volume is replaced inappropriately by high-solute feedings such as skimmed milk. The incidence of hypernatremic dehydration in infantile gastroenteritis is as much as 20% in infants who are bottle fed. It is very low in breast-fed babies. Mortality ranges from 4% to 20%, and seizures are commonly associated with this form of dehydration, leaving permanent sequelae especially in small infants. Hypernatremic dehydration can also occur in individuals with head trauma, tumors, or other lesions of the central nervous system. The etiology of this form of hypernatremic dehydration may be either diabetes insipidus, produced usually through hypothalamic or posterior pituitary dysfunction, or, occasionally, interruption of the neurologically driven thirst mechanisms.

It is important to mention also the hyperosmolar state produced by high blood glucose levels in diabetes mellitus. This condition can cause signs and symptoms similar to those produced by hypernatremic dehydration, but it is often associated with decreased serum concentrations of sodium.

The signs and symptoms of hypernatremic dehydration are produced through the two major compensatory responses, thirst and decreased output of urine, with production of urine of high specific gravity. Signs and symptoms are not usually striking until 10% dehydration has been reached. The effects of hypernatremia itself will also produce particular signs and symptoms, as discussed in Chapter 7. The latter effects are largely neurologic and are caused by the shrinkage of brain cells. As the brain tissue pulls away from the skull, tension on the vessels supplying the brain may produce subarachnoid hemorrhage. Other direct effects of neurologic disturbances include irritability, seizures, motor deficits, and coma. The electroencephalogram may be abnormal, and the cerebrospinal fluid protein concentration can be increased. Other signs and symptoms begin to develop when the ECF volume decreases, but this may not occur until a moribund state is present. Some authorities describe skin texture as "doughy" in hypernatremic dehydration, but this sign is variable and difficult to assess.

The diagnosis of hypernatremic dehydration is based on the finding of an increased serum osmolarity, serum sodium greater than 150 mEq/liter, usually an elevation in chloride, and metabolic acidosis. The dehydration is further confirmed by the history and physical examination.

Treatment of hypernatremic dehydration must be carried out slowly, since there is much evidence that rapid replacement of fluid causes neurologic disturbances and often permanent damage. Replacement in dehydration is accomplished by intravenous administration over a period of 48 to 72 hours, of hypotonic fluids containing dextrose. The repair fluid should contain some solute, since there is evidence that various systems of the body have adjusted to the hypernatremic state, and the return to normal set points is better accomplished when a solute-containing hypotonic fluid is used. It has been recommended by Weil and Bailie (1977) that a solution containing 0.18% sodium chloride and 5% dextrose be administered at the rate of 150 ml/kg/24 hr. (Admission weight is used to determine the total number of milliliters to be given.) Treatment should also be directed at potassium replacement and correction of acidosis. Of course, potassium replacement is started only when the urinary output is satisfactory.

An important aspect of treatment for dehydration should be prevention of the hypernatremic state. Parent teaching can prevent the development of hypernatremia in infants with gastroenteritis, since this condition often develops when high-solute fluids are given to babies with isotonic diarrhea. Many physicians and nurses use handouts indicating the appropriate fluids and foods to be given to children at home, but parents may not understand the instructions, of they may assume, when mixing solutions at home, that larger amounts of salt are better than small amounts.

Hyponatremic dehydration

Hyponatremic dehydration is seen less frequently than isotonic or hypertonic dehydration and is due to loss of solute from the ECF in excess of water loss. Causes of this condition include chronic malnutrition and chronic illness, and there may be no associated symptoms. The acute development of hyponatremic dehydration is symptomatic. It is seen primarily when fluid replacement in a dehydrated individual either is very hypotonic or contains only glucose and is solute free. It is a common assumption that isotonic fluid is being administered when 5% glucose solutions are given. In reality, however, since glucose will quickly enter cells and be metabolized, this solution is hypotonic. Persons with renal disease are particularly prone to develop this form of dehydration. It is necessary to point out that hyponatremia can occur with dehydration, or it can be associated with normal hydration or overhydration. When hypovolemia occurs in conjunction with hyponatremia, the effects on the ECF are primary, since the hypotonicity of the ECF causes excess water to osmose into the cells, thus expanding the ICF and contracting the ECF. As in isotonic dehydration, the symptoms produced by this condition will be cardiovascular and related to the percentage of dehydration. Objective evidence of dehydration will also be present. The skin turgor is greatly decreased, and the skin and mucous membranes are very dry. Oliguria is present and usually very severe. In fact, all the signs of dehydration associated with isotonic loss are present and generally are more severe than with the corresponding percentage of dehydration. Symptoms related to cellular overhydration are usually apparent as well, and they are generally neurologic in origin. Since the cerebrospinal fluid pressure is increased, there are often alterations in the mental state and even convulsions. The differential diagnosis of this condition is therefore complicated.

Treatment of hyponatremic dehydration consists of repair of both the sodium deficit and the volume. The fluid administered should be hyper-

Table 6-2. Physical assessment of dehydration

	HEENT and skin	Cardiovascular	Respiratory	Renal	Gastrointestinal	Neuromuscular
Isotonic dehydration	*Inspection:* Depression of fontanel Skin dry; mucous membranes dry Longitudinal furrows on tongue Sunken abdomen Pallor, cyanosis, mottling of skin *Palpation:* Skin remains in folds when pinched, feels cold and clammy	*Inspection:* Neck veins flat *Palpation:* Pulse deficit Decreased capillary filling *Auscultation:* Heart rate rapid Quality of pulse thready and irregular Blood pressure normal or decreased	*Inspection:* Rate increased because of metabolic acidosis	*Inspection:* Oliguria or anuria Specific gravity: increased	*Palpation:* Pain on deep palpation *Auscultation:* bowel sounds decreased	*Inspection:* Lethargy
Hypertonic dehydration	*Inspection:* Fever caused by increase in basal metabolic rate Nuchal rigidity Shiny appearance of skin Great thirst *Palpation:* "Doughy" feeling of abdominal skin		As above, only milder and with similar percentage of body fluid deficit			*Inspection:* Irritable when aroused; lethargic Muscle twitches, tremors, seizures *Palpation:* Hypertonicity of muscles *Percussion:* Deep tendon reflexes: 3-4+
Hypotonic dehydration	As in isotonic dehydration, only more severe and with similar percentage of body fluid deficit					*Inspection:* Weakness, lethargy, coma *Palpation:* Hypotonicity of muscles *Percussion:* Deep tendon reflexes: 0-1+

tonic, the amount carefully calculated so that the deficit will be repaired, and the water shift into the ECF from the ICF should be taken into account when salt is administered.

Nursing assessment and strategies in dehydration

The history and physical examination of the dehydrated patient are often the only clues to the presence of dehydration in its very early mild stage. The laboratory values may not be significantly altered in isotonic dehydration, and renal changes may be apparent only in moderate to severe dehydration. It is a nursing responsibility to physically assess the patient either in the emergency room or while providing hospital care. The assessment can be meaningful only if the nurses understand the significance of the various alterations that may be present. Table 6-2 summarizes the physical assessment of different body systems and the findings in dehydration.

The care of the dehydrated patient is challenging and must be based on an excellent understanding of the pathophysiology involved. Offering a patient Gatorade, for example, may be an excellent way to repair fluid loss but is certainly not appropriate in all types of dehydration. The nurse must be able to independently measure and calculate fluid losses and gains and is often in a position to choose appropriate oral fluids, as well as to assume responsibility for the administration of intravenous fluids and the care of the patient during this time. Furthermore, patient teaching plays a crucial role in care and is usually the major responsibility of the nurse. Continuous assessment of the dehydration and electrolyte abnormalities and of the response to treatment must be carried out by nurses caring for the patient. Therefore the nursing care plan must be modified as the patient's condition changes and must reflect the changing data base. The goals of nursing care must be based on the assessment of the patient. The major problem areas we have discussed with regard to dehydration relate to circulatory collapse, either imminent or real, renal and splanchnic perfusion, tonicity disturbances, and electrolyte and acid-base abnormalities. The signs and symptoms produced by these various alterations must be assessed frequently by the nurse who is caring for the dehydrated patient.

CASE STUDY • INFANT WITH HYPERNATREMIC DEHYDRATION

A 5-month-old infant developed hypernatremic dehydration as the result of gastroenteritis. The infant had previously been well and had received the usual immunizations and well-baby checkups. He was bottle-fed with Similac and was developing normally, weighing 6.8 kg (15 lb). The parents were very young, and this baby was their first child. When taking the history the nurse observed that both parents seemed apprehensive of all medical personnel and procedures, and the mother confessed that she had felt too intimidated to call her pediatrician's office when the baby first became ill. Three days before admission the baby developed a fever and became extremely irritable. He vomited several times and became lethargic in the evening, refusing to drink more than a few ounces of formula. During the next day he developed a fever of 40° C (104° F) and began to have profuse green liquid diarrhea. He appeared very thirsty, taking formula eagerly but then vomiting most of it later. His mother gave him aspirin and urged formula, but the baby took very little, continued to have a high fever, and cried incessantly. Early in the morning of the day of admission the mother went to the emergency room of the local hospital with the baby, who had suffered a seizure at home.

On examination in the emergency room, the vital signs and laboratory findings were as follows:

Vital signs	*Laboratory data*
Weight: 6.1 kg	White blood cell count: 4300
Blood pressure: 90/60	Lymphocytes, 40%; polymorphonuclear
Temperature: 58.1° C (104.6° F)	leukocytes, 50%; eosinophils, 1%;
Pulse: 168 beats/min	monocytes, 8%; basophils, 1%
Respirations: 45/min	Hematocrit: 58%
	Hemoglobin: 16 gm
	Na^+: 150 mEq/liter
	K^+: 5.8 mEq/liter
	Cl^-: 110 mEq/liter
	pH: 7.26
	Serum osmolarity: 302 mOsm
	Urinalysis: pH 4.0; specific gravity
	1.030; no cells or casts

PHYSICAL ASSESSMENT

General findings: Flushed, very lethargic infant with sunken eyes, poor skin turgor, depressed fontanel, dry mouth and skin, dry diaper, no stools at present.

Eyes, ears, and nose: Baby cries without apparent reason.

Neck: Full range of motion, trachea midline, neck veins flat (above clavicle) when infant is both supine and sitting up.

Head: Anterior fontanel depressed; normocephalic; circumference, 43 cm.

Throat: Slightly injected, with no tonsillar hypertrophy. Mucous membranes dry; tongue furrowed.

Thorax: Respirations rapid with regular rate, deep inspirations. Chest clear to auscultation and percussion. Equal expansion and diaphragmatic excursion; no retractions.

Cardiovascular system: Heart rate rapid and thready, with radial pulses

barely palpable. Point of maximal impulse (PMI) at fifth intercostal
space in midclavicular line. No murmurs.

Abdomen: Soft, sunken; no palpable masses.

Genitalia: Within normal limits (WNL); diaper dry.

Joints and muscles: Good range of motion in all joints, but client irritable when aroused and does not like being handled at present
time. Muscle mass normal for age, but motor activity minimal at
this time.

Neurologic findings: Client is apparently postictal. Can be aroused
fairly easily but is extremely lethargic and sleepy. Reflexes 3+
bilaterally (knee, triceps, biceps, Achilles tendon). Babinski's reflex
positive. Sensations intact to touch and pinprick, but responses
somewhat sluggish. Pupillary reflex normal, but pupils appear
somewhat dilated. Cranial nerves not tested.

TREATMENT

This baby was apparently suffering 10% dehydration by weight (and as
indicated in the physical examination) and was in early hypovolemic
shock. Furthermore, the serum concentrations of sodium, osmolarity
values, and other symptoms indicated hypernatremia. He was admitted
to the hospital, and hydration was begun intravenously with 5% dextrose
in 0.16% saline solution, in the amounts indicated:

1. Maintenance: stool loss = 238 ml, IWL = 354 ml, renal loss = 340
ml (total of 932 ml/24 hr)
2. Repair: 680 ml/36 hr

He recovered completely, slowly beginning oral feedings, and suffered
no apparent neurologic sequelae. The nurses caring for this family were
able to teach the parents certain aspects of well-baby care and to reestab-
lish their trust in health professionals.

OVERHYDRATION

Overhydration is a clinical state characterized by an excess of ECF.
Like dehydration, it is a sign of underlying pathology, not a disease entity
in itself. Most commonly, overhydration is associated with renal or cardiovascular disease. It may be seen when isotonic saline solution is administered to patients in excessive amounts, since intravenous saline solution
will remain trapped in the plasma compartment and must be excreted
largely through the kidneys. ECF excess may also be present when plasma
proteins are decreased, as might occur in severe malnutrition or in liver
or kidney disease. The decreased colloid osmotic pressure of the blood
causes more fluid to be retained in the interstitial fluid (edema). The
body can become overhydrated during surgical stress as well, primarily
as the result of excessive ADH stimulation. Overhydration may also be
the result of shifts of interstitial fluid into the plasma and consequent
hypervolemia (increased plasma volume).

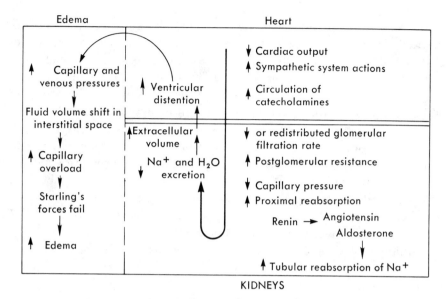

Fig. 6-3. Pathogenesis of cardiac edema. (From Groër, M. E., and Shekleton, M. E.: Basic pathophysiology: a conceptual approach, St. Louis, 1979, The C. V. Mosby Co.)

From the above description it is apparent that overhydration may occur as an overall accumulation of excess ECF or as a separate excess in either the plasma or interstitial fluid compartment.

In cardiac disease an overall excess of fluid in both the vascular and interstitial spaces occurs. The etiology of this fluid accumulation is diagramed in Fig. 6-3. Heart failure is the primary cause of the fluid problem and may be either "forward" or "backward" failure. In forward heart failure the heart becomes inadequate as a pump; it does not propel the blood from the left ventricle with sufficient ejection force or with sufficient stroke volume. The cause may be an inherent weakness in the myocardium itself, such as occurs frequently after myocardial infarction damage, or it may be an increased resistance to the ejection of the blood from the heart during systole. The latter cause is present in hypertension, in which the total peripheral resistance is increased, causing the cardiac output to increase in a compensatory manner through myocardial hypertrophy. A point is reached at which further hypertrophy of the heart does not produce greater systolic ejection force but is rather a pathologic stretching of heart muscle fibers and dilation of the heart. When this point is reached, the heart becomes a less effective pump. After systole, the volume of blood remaining in the left ventricle is greater than normal, and the resulting increased end systolic volume causes increased ventricular pressure. As with any open system, the pressure in one chamber as it increases will cause a backing up of pressure within tubes that are connected to the chamber. With regard to the left ventricle, the open communication is with the left atrium and pulmonary veins. By the simple laws of physics it is apparent that if enough pressure is present, the entire heart will become involved, since it is an open system of communication through the pulmonary vessels. The pressure is hydrostatic and will result in filtration of fluid into the lungs in excess of that reabsorbed, and pulmonary edema becomes manifested at this point. Furthermore, the right heart becomes involved, and "backward" heart failure results. In this condition the right heart cannot adequately pump against the increasing pulmonary resistance. The fluid pressure rises in the right heart chambers and causes increasing pressure in the venous side of the circulation. Venous and capillary engorgement is the result.

In both right and left heart failure, the total ECF volume increases, often dramatically. Of course, with forward failure the major symptoms are related to the pulmonary congestion. However, a significant increase in the ECF volume occurs as the result of renal response to the decreased kidney perfusion that is present when the heart is not able to adequately pump out enough blood. The kidneys interpret the resultant decreased blood flow and renal hypoxia as a volume depletion. Instead of the normal physiologic body water regulation, a pathophysiologic response becomes evident. The kidneys, to conserve body water, release renin, and through the renin-angiotensin-aldosterone mechanism, sodium and water reabsorption in the distal convoluted tubule (DCT) is greatly enhanced. The ECF becomes expanded as the result of this normally helpful compensatory mechanism. However, in forward failure the expansion of the ECF only increases the load on the heart and the work it must perform. Therefore the weakened, failing heart will become even more overburdened, as seen in Fig. 6-3. The pulmonary congestion and edema will be further perpetuated.

Backward failure causes a similar response by the kidney, through venous congestion. The venous and capillary engorgement increases the hydrostatic pressure in the capillary bed, disrupting the Starling forces so that excessive filtration occurs and leads to interstitial edema. Furthermore the tissues become hypoxic because of the vascular stasis of venous, deoxygenated blood. The kidney becomes subject to stagnant hypoxia, which triggers renin release with subsequent sodium and water retention. The excessive filtration of blood into the interstitial spaces will also reduce blood volume initially, and this reduction may contribute to sodium retention through aldosterone release. The exact pathophysiologic process by which sodium and water retention occurs in congestive heart failure has not been clearly elucidated, but these mechanisms are widely accepted as probable causes.

Edema

Nurses encounter patients with edema both within the hospital setting and in the community. It is important to be able to recognize edema and to assess the patient carefully. Pitting edema is interstitial fluid excess that accumulates in dependent parts of the body, such as the legs and feet, or in the sacral area of a patient on best rest. It is characterized by the appearance of a depression, or "pit," in the skin when the area is gently pushed by the examiner's finger. The depression, which only gradually returns to the normal state, is caused by the physical pressure of the finger as it pushes away fluid and displaces it momentarily. The edematous patient may initially give the false appearance of good health and nutrition, but closer examination may indicate cachectic wasting obscured by the edematous tissues. Body weight may actually increase significantly while the patient is in negative nitrogen balance and is undergoing muscular wasting. The cardiac patient develops pitting edema because of right heart failure, ineffective circulating blood volume, and resultant renal retention of sodium and water. The patient with kidney disease may develop edema when there is inadequate excretion of water and electrolytes through the urine, as in renal failure, or when albumin is lost through the urine with resultant hypoalbuminemia, as in nephrotic syndrome. Another important cause of edema is hepatic disease, particularly cirrhosis of the liver. The result is an accumulation of ECF within the abdominal cavity, leading to a great increase in abdominal girth. This accumulation of fluid is called ascites. The pathogenesis is through portal vein obstruction caused by hepatic scarring and enlargement, which inhibit blood flow through the portal vein. The hydrostatic pressure therefore increases and causes plasma fluid to leak through the intestinal capillaries or liver sinusoids into the abdominal cavity. Commonly also, the increased abdominal pressure caused by fluid accumulation results in obstructed outflow from the femoral veins draining the lower extremities. This increased hydrostatic pressure is reflected back into the capillaries and causes the formation of further edema in the legs.

Edema is seen in many other conditions as well and may be localized or general, and pitting or nonpitting. There may be periorbital edema, for example, in a patient experiencing an allergic reaction that causes the release of histamine. This biogenic amine increases capillary permeability, and thus filtration is favored over reabsorption in the capillaries. Other inflammatory processes may be associated with edema because of similar vascular effects of the mediators of the inflammatory response. For example, when a burn damages or destroys blood vessels, edema fluid forms. Another factor that contributes to edema formation is alteration in the integrity of the lymphatic system. If the lymphatic vessels become obstructed through trauma or infection, there is an overall tendency toward excessive filtration and protein leak into the interstitial fluid, which are unopposed by lymphatic drainage of protein and excess fluid. Certain drugs, such as oral contraceptives and glucocorticoids, can cause edema through effects on renal sodium reabsorption.

Pulmonary edema can be a dramatic, life-threatening condition or, less commonly, can develop insidiously when ECF actually accumulates within the very loose pulmonary interstitium and alveolar spaces. This accumulation impairs oxygen and carbon dioxide exchange and produces a state of hypercapnia and eventually hypoxemia. The patient with pulmonary edema becomes exhausted by the work of breathing, and of course the increased work results in an increased oxygen and nutritional demand, further burdening the patient and creating a vicious cycle. The patient is orthopneic, tachycardiac, and cyanotic, and bubbling rales may be heard throughout the lung fields. A cough is present and produces blood-tinged sputum. The patient hyperventilates but usually is not able to compensate for the respiratory acidosis, and oxygen is usually required. Often there are no signs of interstitial edema in other areas of the body if the congestive heart failure is purely left-sided, forward failure. The overall ECF volume increases in pulmonary edema because of renal retention of sodium and water, which, of course, will further perpetuate the development of pulmonary edema. Therefore an important therapeutic approach for such a patient consists of diuretic therapy, which is also a major approach to the treatment of patients with interstitial edema, as previously described. Sodium restriction (usually less than 3 gm/24 hr) also decreases the fluid retention, and in heart failure the administration of digitalis preparations increases myocardial strength in the failing heart and thus enhances cardiac output. Another important aspect of care is fluid restriction, particularly if the patient is suffering from acute dilutive hyponatremia, caused in many cases by inadequate kidney function and by excess water retention that produces a state of water intoxication. Rest

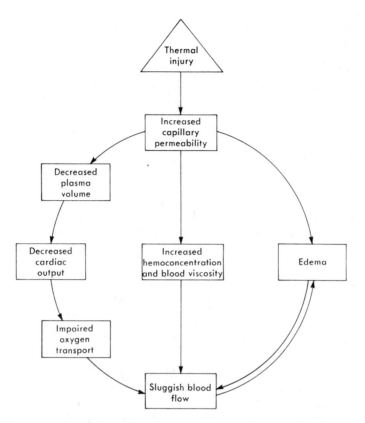

Fig. 6-4. In severe burns, capillary permeability is increased, allowing protein-rich plasma to leak from vascular to intravascular spaces and causing edema, hemoconcentration, and decrease in cardiac output. (From Groër, M. E., and Shekleton, M. E.: Basic pathophysiology: a conceptual approach, St. Louis, 1979, The C. V. Mosby Co.)

is the fourth cornerstone of treatment of edema. Its benefits can be marked and may actually prevent the development of congestive heart failure in a patient at risk. Rest may produce an isotonic diuresis that will be greatly beneficial to the edematous patient.

Edema accompanying a severe burn represents a loss of vascular fluid into the injured, inflamed interstitium, with a drop in vascular volume and an expansion of interstitial volume. The pathophysiology of burn edema is illustrated in Fig. 6-4. This kind of edema represents third-space edema, in which fluid is lost into a compartment of body fluid and is basically unavailable for exchange with other fluid compartments.

Furthermore, fluids are continuously lost through the burned skin by IWL, which may be ten times the normal loss. Burned patients experience a rapid hypermetabolism that increases heat production tremendously, and the burned skin is an ineffective barrier for heat containment. The loss of fluid in edema and increased IWL can be so great that the major problem the patient experiences in the first 2 days after receiving a burn is the danger of decreased plasma volume leading to hypovolemic shock. The cardiac output falls, and widespread SNS activity is present as a compensatory mechanism. This shock state is present in an individual who may be grossly edematous from the burn. Another effect of the early fluid shift and edema is hemoconcentration, which occurs as excess plasma is lost from the blood, thus concentrating the formed elements of the blood (leukocytes, erythrocytes, and platelets). Since the viscosity of the blood increases, and because of vascular damage and metabolic acidosis, the burned patient is at risk for the development of thrombi and emboli. An additional fluid and electrolyte problem is hyperkalemia during the first phase after the burn. Hyponatremia may also accompany the hyperkalemia. The increase in serum concentration of potassium results from the damage and death of the burned cells. Since potassium is the major intracellular cation, the destruction of large numbers of cells will result in a release of potassium into the ECF. Hyponatremia may develop as a result of excessive sodium loss into cells. Burned cells also show injury-related changes in enzymatic function, and the Na^+-K^+ pump is inhibited by a lack of ATP and overwhelmed by the increased permeability of the damaged membrane.

The fluid, electrolyte, and acid-base problems of the burned patient change remarkably in the second phase of recovery from a burn injury. After about 2 days a second fluid shift occurs in which edema fluid is remobilized from the burn site back into the vascular compartment. This shift occurs because of the recovery of the vascular endothelium, which will then permit the normal Starling forces to operate. At this point plasma volume will become expanded and dilutive effects manifested. Diuresis will also occur, as well as hypokalemia, which can be very severe. It results from the potassium excretion that has occurred through the kidneys during the transient period of hyperkalemia, as well as from the reabsorption of potassium by the recovering cells. It is necessary to observe the patient for diuresis after the first 48 hours to determine whether fluid remobilization is occurring, so that appropriate measures can be taken to avoid hypokalemia and fluid overload.

Obviously the treatment of the burned patient during the first 48 hours is aimed at avoiding hypovolemic shock. Large amounts of fluid are needed to balance the IWL and to replace the fluid lost into the interstitium. The choice of fluid is based on the fluid and electrolyte composition of the loss. IWL is replaced by solutions of 5% dextrose in water, whereas vascular loss into the burn is replaced by isotonic saline solution with additional colloid added to compensate for the protein loss into the edema fluid. A common solution used is Brook's formula, which is composed of colloid, electrolytes, and dextrose according to the following calculations:

> Dextrose, 5%, in water = 2000 ml in adults
> Normal saline solution = Kilograms of body weight × % burn × 115 ml
> Colloid = Kilograms of body weight × % burn × 0.5 ml

This formula is corrected for the child; IWL is replaced by 5% dextrose in water in amounts ranging from 150 ml/kg in a 2-year-old child to 50 ml/kg in an 8-year-old child. This intravenous solution is altered during the second 24 hours, and only half of the colloid and saline solution is administered during the second 24 hours, although the replacement of IWL remains the same.

Nursing responsibilities in the care of the burned patient must be carried out with a full understanding of the physiology and pathophysiology that are operating. Assessment of the body systems during the first phase is aimed at early detection of the major problems of hypovolemia, hyperkalemia and hyponatremia, and metabolic acidosis. Respiratory acidosis or alkalosis can also be present in these patients because of burn-related respiratory damage (in acidosis) or because of hyperventilation resulting from anxiety (in alkalosis). Nursing measures that will promote the fluid balance and comfort of the patient include humidification of the environment to prevent excessive IWL, safety measures to prevent infection, encouragement of fluid and nutrient intake when possible, continuous assessment of intake and output, and other evaluations of fluid and electrolyte balance.

Water intoxication

Water intoxication is a situation in which the total body water (TBW) is expanded, either because of excessive water ingestion over loss or because of inappropriate ADH secretion. The net effect is dilution of the ECF, with resulting osmosis of water into cells and consequent expansion of ICF. Some aspects of this state resemble hyponatremic dehydration (previously discussed), but it must be remembered that in this con-

Table 6-3. Conditions resulting in the syndrome of inappropriate ADH

Mechanism	Condition
Increased ADH secretion	Stress (e.g., surgery, heat)
	Neoplasms
	Guillain-Barré syndrome
	Infections
	Drugs (e.g., chlorpropamide [Diabinese], cyclophosphamide [Cytoxan], thiothixene [Navane])
	Endocrinopathies
	Idiopathic conditions
Ectopic ADH production	Hormone-secreting carcinomas
Potentiation of effect	Diabinese

dition there is overhydration, although hyponatremia is a consequence of the water excess. Table 6-3 lists the conditions that may be associated with the syndrome of inappropriate ADH secretion (SIADH). Increased ADH secretion results in inappropriate retention of water through the action of ADH on the collecting ducts. This retention will decrease the urine output and dilute the ECF. Great physiologic stress may be a cause of this syndrome and may lead to water intoxication. For example, the syndrome can be seen in trauma, as is most evidenced by the postoperative occurrence of water intoxication, since surgical stress is a potent stimulator of ADH. SIADH is particularly frequent in aged individuals who have undergone major surgery, usually becoming manifested between 24 and 48 hours after the surgery. The exact neurologic pathways through which body injury or surgical incision stimulates hypothalamic production of ADH are not known. The effects are transient, but in severely debilitated or seriously ill patients the effects of water intoxication can be severe. The symptoms of water intoxication caused by SIADH include weight gain, excretion of urine of high specific gravity, decreased urine output (less than 500 ml/24 hr), and hypotonic serum, which is reflected in decreases in serum concentrations of sodium and chloride, as well as in dilutive effects on the plasma proteins. The subjective findings usually are indicative of neurologic impairment caused by osmotic swelling. Table 6-4 shows the physical assessment of a patient with water intoxication. Gradations of severity exist, but most surgical patients exhibit no pathologic effects because hyponatremia and water overload are not severe. All surgical patients should nevertheless be assessed by the nurse for signs of water intoxication.

Table 6-4. Physical assessment of water intoxication

	Head, eyes, ears, nose, throat	Cardiovascular system	Gastro-intestinal system	Respiratory system	Integu-mentary system	Neuromuscular system	Renal system
Inspection	Decreased lacrimation and salivation Late signs: papilledema, blurred vision, projectile vomiting, headache	Venous congestion	Watery diarrhea Nausea and vomiting			Muscle cramps Disorientation Restlessness Muscle twitching	Oliguria
Palpation		Distention of peripheral veins and neck veins			Pitting of skin during pressure	Muscle weakness	
Percussion						Increased deep tendon reflexes (early) Decreased deep tendon reflexes (late)	
Auscultation		Increased heart rate and blood pressure		Hyperpnea Rales Other symptoms of pulmonary edema			

7

Sodium imbalance

The taste or desire for salt is present in mammals and appears to be a mechanism for controlling the intake of salt. When rats are given the choice of drinking different solutions containing salt, they prefer salty solutions, in a concentration of up to about 1%. Salt receptors are present in man in the taste buds of the tongue. There are individual taste cells for four different taste sensations: salty, sour, sweet, and bitter. An individual "salty" taste cell is fired and transmits messages to the central nervous system when salt is present in food or drink. Other taste cells may be weakly sensitive to salt and vice versa, but the salty taste cells are the most sensitive, or most easily stimulated by salt. It is interesting from an evolutionary and behavioral perspective to examine the obvious preference civilized groups have for salt. Excessive salting of the food, far beyond the requirements of body tonicity, is typical of the average American. There is evidence that this desire for salty food is, in fact, harmful and may contribute to hypertension. Yet most of us describe our food as tasteless and bland without the addition of sodium chloride. According to Dethier, the salt receptor cells are an evolutionary heritage and represent cells originally used by our primitive ancestors as environmental sensors, acting primarily to protect the organism. Their general irritability to salt stimuli is thought to have been protective. Some so-called salt receptors exist in the human eye and on the wings of flies, where their function is dubious. The retention of salt receptors on the tongue is probably an evolutionary advantage, however, since in cases of hyponatremia or in disorders of the adrenal gland, such as Addison's disease, salt craving exists in humans. These cells may represent a part of a physiologic feedback loop that controls ECF osmolarity. However, cultural and behavioral factors appear to be almost as important as our true need for sodium chloride in states of health, and even in primitive cultures the salty taste is considered pleasant.

CONTROL OF SODIUM

Sodium balance is intimately tied to water balance, which was discussed in Chapter 2. The effects of volume deficits or excesses were described in Chapter 6. This chapter now presents the more detailed aspects of sodium balance and imbalance, without repetition of concepts already discussed.

The compartmentalization of sodium is diagramed in Fig. 7-1. It can be seen that most of the total body sodium is extracellular and that most of this extracellular sodium is contained within the bone. This sodium is largely nonexchangeable with the ECF sodium, except for about 14%. Another large sodium compartment consists of cartilage and connective tissue; thus only 40% of the total body sodium is in the plasma and tissue fluid. Nevertheless, sodium is the major cation of the ECF, existing at a concentration of 136 to 144 mEq/liter in the blood plasma.

Sodium balance is regulated largely through renal tubular reabsorption. Thus sodium in the plasma is normally filtered at the glomerulus and reabsorbed according to the body's needs at the proximal and distal convoluted tubules. Most of the sodium reabsorption is obligatory and occurs at the proximal convoluted tubule (PCT). This sodium reabsorption is not affected by the hormone aldosterone. Aldosterone increases sodium reabsorption at the distal convoluted tubule (DCT) and to a minor degree at the collecting ducts. The effects of aldosterone are to increase both sodium reabsorption and K^+ and H^+ excretion. Thus, when excess aldosterone is present, as in certain aldosterone-secreting adenomas, there is a resultant increase in sodium reabsorption, coupled with excess potassium loss leading to hypokalemia, and an excess H^+ excretion leading to metabolic alkalosis. The cells respond to hypokalemia by increased

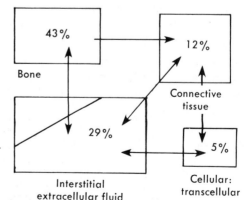

Fig. 7-1. Body sodium compartments.

efflux of potassium, and electrical requirements therefore dictate increased H^+ influx into the cells to the point where the cells become acidotic. It is important to note that aldosterone affects K^+ and H^+ secretion only if sodium is present in the distal tubular filtrate and adequate distal tubular flow is present. Aldosterone secretion was previously described in Chapters 2 and 3. Briefly, the major stimuli for release of aldosterone from the adrenal cortex are the action of the renin-angiotensin system, secretion of adrenocorticotropic hormone (ACTH), and hyperkalemia. The latter two stimuli act through direct effects on the adrenal gland, where formation of the hormone is enhanced. Another probably existing hormone controls sodium balance and is elusively known as the "third factor," the glomerular filtration rate (GFR), representing the "first" factor and aldosterone the "second" factor. The third factor is *natriuretic*, or salt wasting, in action. It increases sodium excretion when there has been an increase in ECF volume from sodium retention. In other words, it overcomes the aldosterone effects of increased sodium and water retention and is seen in persons who have apparently adapted to high levels of aldosterone over several days through release of the third factor. Thus the major stimulus for the third factor is hypervolemia, and its action is to correct the hypervolemia through salt wasting and water diuresis.

Since Na^+ is the major cation of the ECF, it exerts the greatest proportion of ECF osmolarity. Osmolarity of the plasma is roughly determined by measuring the serum sodium in milliequivalents per liter and then multiplying this value by 2. The product is the milliosmoles per liter of plasma water. Thus it is apparent that the regulation of the extracellular sodium plays a great role in the regulation of ECF volume because of sodium's osmotic influence. Conversely, decreases or increases in plasma volume will stimulate or inhibit aldosterone release, which will regulate sodium reabsorption in such a manner as to restore the plasma volume to normal. There is also evidence that excessive or decreased volume of the interstitial fluid space, through an as-yet-unknown mechanism, depresses or stimulates aldosterone release. Another point of interest is that plasma sodium values play only a minor role in aldosterone release and sodium reabsorption, and plasma volume balance overrides any effects of hyponatremia or hypernatremia. In a person with hypernatremic dehydration (pp. 142 to 144) there would be an increase in sodium reabsorption and a corresponding expansion of plasma volume, even though this would raise the levels of total body sodium. Another interesting phenomenon is the inability of a person with hyponatremia to form an alkaline urine to compensate for hyperventilation. In this case sodium reabsorption takes precedence over bicarbonate excretion. It is important to remember this fact because hyponatremia and alkalosis can occur together in prolonged vomiting, and yet the patient may continue to form an acid urine.

SODIUM IMBALANCES

An understanding of the physiologic effects of altered ECF and total body sodium is best achieved with a background knowledge of cell membrane phenomena, as presented in Chapter 3. Briefly, the reason that sodium does not easily enter cells is the great impermeability of the cellular membrane. This changes only when the cell is stimulated to depolarize, and the result is a cell membrane that is transiently freely permeable to sodium. The ion moves down its electrical and concentration gradient into the cell, making the cell membrane more positively charged, as compared to the outside. If sufficiently depolarized, the cell reaches threshold and fires an action potential. Thus the effects of sodium imbalance relate to (1) osmotic consequences of alterations in sodium and (2) cell membrane irritability.

Hyponatremia

Table 7-1 summarizes the various possible causes of hyponatremia, which is defined as a serum concentration of sodium of less than 136 mEq/liter. Since this is a measure of the *concentration* of sodium, hyponatremia may occur either when there is a *net loss of sodium* or when there is a *net gain of water.* Hyponatremia, whatever the cause, usually implies a drop in plasma and ECF osmolarity. However, this does not

Table 7-1. Causes of hyponatremia

Net sodium loss	Net water excess
Kidney diseases	Syndrome of inappropriate ADH secretion (SIADH)
Addison's disease	
Gastrointestinal losses	Increase of water over solute intake, when renal mechanisms are not functioning properly
Increased sweating	
Diuretics	
Interruption of Na^+-K^+ pump with decreased cell K^+ and decreased serum Na^+	Hyperaldosteronism
	Diabetic ketoacidosis
Use of diuretics combined with low-sodium diet	Oliguria caused by renal failure
	Psychogenic polydipsia
Metabolic acidosis	

occur in diabetes, which is associated with high blood glucose levels. Often there are a drop in serum concentrations of sodium and an increased plasma volume caused by the osmotic effects of glucose. For serum osmolarity to be unaffected in hyponatremia, additional osmotically active particles that compensate for the loss of sodium must be present.

Net sodium deficits. When there is an overall net loss of body sodium, the physiologic compensatory response to this decrease is water excretion through the kidneys so as to maintain the serum osmolarity at normal levels. This is the earliest response to sodium deficit. Later in the process, however, the body favors preservation of the blood and interstitial volume, with the consequence that the sodium in the ECF becomes more and more dilute (i.e., hyponatremia is recognizable by laboratory values and by clinical signs and symptoms). Furthermore, in this type of sodium deficit, there is an overall decrease in ECF volume, which is in contrast with those disorders in which water excess acts to dilute the ECF sodium and expand the ECF compartment. Naturally the symptoms of these two forms of hyponatremia are very different. In the former we see signs of vascular collapse, imminent or real, and in the latter there can be all the signs of overhydration, such as heart failure, dyspnea, and edema.

In hyponatremia associated with net sodium deficit and contraction of the ECF, there are several diagnostic clues to the identification of the condition. By the time the patient is truly dehydrated, the picture will be the same as in hyponatremic dehydration, as discussed in Chapter 6. As the state develops, there is decreased secretion of sweat, saliva, and urine. The specific gravity of the urine is low, the blood urea nitrogen level often increases and, of course, the electrolyte study shows hyponatremia and hypochloremia, which develop as the kidneys begin to conserve water in the presence of continuing low sodium levels. It is important to obtain the history of the development of symptoms so that the etiology of the hyponatremia can be established. The physical assessment of the patient will reveal general apathy, lethargy and weakness, weight loss, signs of decreased blood volume such as a drop in blood pressure, postural hypotension, weak fast pulse with a decreased aortic second sound, decreased peripheral venous filling, coolness of the skin, decreased skin turgor, absence of thirst, and a drop in core body temperature. Most of these symptoms relate directly to the decreased ECF volume.

The effects of decreased ECF sodium on cellular irritability and conductivity are also apparent. Since the gradient for diffusion of sodium into cells is less when the cells are stimulated, increased stimulation strength and a longer time will be needed for cells to sufficiently depolarize before reaching threshold and firing. Of course, the cells most profoundly affected include nerve and muscle, which accounts for the central nervous system effects of hyponatremia and muscle weakness. Other signs of decreased irritability of the nervous system include a decline in the strength of the deep tendon reflexes, the appearance of a positive Babinski's reflex, and even palsy and paralysis. In patients with severe but chronic hyponatremia, the personality changes reflect excessive irritability, confusion, and aggression. This latter effect may be the result of osmotic swelling of the brain that would occur in the face of declining ECF osmolarity. Muscle twitches, tremors, and cramping may also be part of the clinical picture, particularly when the deficit develops rapidly. The hemoglobin and hematocrit values may reflect hemoconcentration, which will increase the viscosity and sluggishness of the blood and, combined with the usual peripheral vasoconstriction and hypoxia, will consequently also increase the possibility of thrombus and embolus formation.

After the problem has been identified, the treatment is aimed at restoring both the volume deficit and the sodium deficit by administering salt-containing IV fluids. The osmotic strength of the solution is determined by the degree of sodium deficit and the condition of the patient. A hypertonic solution may be administered, but not too rapidly. The amount of sodium needed to repair the deficit is determined by subtracting the plasma sodium concentration from the normal desired values, and the total volume of body water (TBW) is determined by the percentage value of the body weight (in kilograms), which is 60% in adults. The resulting figure represents the total amount of sodium (in milliequivalents) needed to restore the body fluids to normal sodium concentration and osmotic strength. Hypertonic saline solution, 3% to 5%, usually administered over 48 hours, is considered the best form of treatment. Many patients will also require plasma or plasma expanders, since there is always the threat of hypovolemic shock in sodium and water deficit.

The nursing assessments and strategies are similar to those in patients with hyponatremic dehydration. Clearly, the major concerns of the nurse are to help correct the problem and to avoid the occurrence of shock. Excellent assessment of the patient, from the primary contact throughout the treatment period, is thus a nursing responsibility.

Net water excesses. Hyponatremia may also develop in the patient because of a large excess of ECF water that may occur as a consequence of the conditions listed in Table 7-1. These conditions result in dilutive effects on all formed blood elements and on all plasma and interstitial fluid solutes. Such a state is best described as water intoxication (Chapter 6). The clinical syndrome associated with dilutive hyponatremia is vastly different from the one just described, in which there is a net sodium deficit accompanied by a water deficit. Therefore a patient should never receive a hypertonic saline solution on the basis of the serum concentration of sodium alone. Imagine the results of infusion of perhaps several hundred milliequivalents of sodium into the ECF of a patient who is hyponatremic because of water intoxication. The infused sodium, being osmotically active, will further increase the water concentration of the ECF and thus perpetuate the pathophysiologic changes. The great importance of the history and physical examination is obvious, since the conditions and the treatments are so dissimilar. The physical assessment of the hyponatremic patient usually reveals weight gain, hypervolemic signs and symptoms, edema, low hematocrit and hemoglobin values, and hypoalbuminemia. The urine volume is normal or excessive, and there is often a normal specific gravity. Cardiovascular evaluation may show peripheral venous distention, a rapid, bounding pulse, elevated blood pressure, murmurs, and loud and crisp S_1 and S_2 heart sounds. A gallop rhythm may also be present. Weakness and hyporeflexia may be present, but muscle cramping during exercise is frequently present (stoker's cramps).

The treatment of hyponatremia associated with water excess is aimed at reducing the ECF and ICF volume excesses. Treatment of the primary disease process, if it is possible, obviously plays an important part in the therapeutic approach. Additionally, water restriction and diuretics are frequently used. However, the latter drugs are given with care because hyponatremia may develop as the result of diuretic therapy. Titration of the serum concentration of sodium in certain patients may be done by combining a diuretic and hypertonic saline solution, particularly in the syndrome of inappropriate ADH secretion (SIADH). In this approach the diuretic induces both a water loss and a sodium loss. The sodium lost is replaced in the smaller volume of hypertonic solution that is administered. An eventual state of sodium and water balance can then be achieved.

Hypernatremia

Hypernatremia is a state in which the ECF concentration of sodium is greater than 150 mEq/liter. Chapter 6 described the condition of hypernatremic dehydration in some detail. Therefore only certain aspects of hypernatremia will be reviewed here.

Etiology. Table 7-2 lists the most common causes of hypernatremia—those associated with net water deficit or net sodium excess in a manner

Table 7-2. Common causes of hypernatremia

Net water deficit	Net sodium excess
Water deprivation	Imbibing of large amounts of concentrated
Urea diuresis	salt solutions, especially in infants
Greatly increased insensible	Iatrogenic administration of hypertonic saline
water loss (IWL)	solutions parenterally
Disorders in which thirst is either	
absent or not perceived	
Nephrogenic diabetes insipidus	

similar to the pathophysiology of hyponatremia, except in the opposite direction.

The physiologic responses to hypernatremia include maximum stimulation of ADH for the purpose of conserving as much water as possible through renal reabsorption. The result is the excretion, in small amounts, of a urine with a high specific gravity. Another interesting effect of hypernatremia is fever, which is presumed to be caused by an excessively high metabolic rate as the sodium gradient into the cells from the ECF is enhanced. For cell membrane potential and size to be maintained, the Na^+-K^+ pump must operate at maximum efficiency. This causes an increased demand for ATP production that, if met, will result in greater heat production by cells and thus a rise in the core body temperature. Regardless of the etiology of hypernatremia, the result is increased plasma and interstitial osmotic pressure. This hyperosmolarity will result in osmosis of cellular water into the ECF compartment, and the cells will shrink. Crenation of cells interrupts most of the physiologic processes, since all cells require a fluid cytoplasm and are dependent on proper shape and size for function. There is evidence that morphologic configuration of the erythrocytes, for example, results in interruption of normal sodium transport (Groër and Omachi, 1974).

Particularly affected are neurons of the central nervous system. Two factors influence these cells in hypernatremia: (1) the sodium gradient itself and its effect on irritability and conduction and (2) the osmotic shrinkage of the cells. The former effect is related to the increased sodium entry into the cell when the excitable cells are stimulated to fire. Depolarization will be faster, and less stimulus strength will be required to sufficiently depolarize the cell to threshold. The cells are more highly irritable because of this phenomenon. The relevant symptoms of hypernatremia were described in Chapter 6. It is necessary to point out that the predictable electrical events may be overshadowed by the cell volume changes. Thus muscle weakness is often a major sign of hypernatremia, and this is not what one might expect to see, based on the electrical events.

Osmotic shrinkage of cells is, in a sense, a protective mechanism, since the brain's osmoreceptors are stimulated when the ECF osmolarity rises. This stimulation results in the sensation of thirst and the stimulation of ADH. In normal persons the rise in ECF concentration of sodium will be quickly alleviated through these two mechanisms. Thus we do not often see hypernatremia in previously well persons, even if they have a large insensible water loss (IWL), which could theoretically cause hypernatremia. However, in a small infant, who is unable to communicate thirst and who is given salt-containing fluids to replace the IWL, hypernatremia can easily occur. Hypernatremia can be associated with dehydration caused by net water deficit, as discussed in Chapter 6, or it can be present in association with net sodium gain, which causes an expansion of the ECF. Again, as in hyponatremia, the symptoms of these two possible conditions differ, since there is, in one case, dehydration and, in the other, overhydration. A net sodium gain may not be reflected in plasma osmolarity, however. Because of the efficient aldosterone-mediated mechanism in the DCT, and also because of ADH action, a net salt load, which will be associated with water retention, will inhibit aldosterone and ADH, causing a sodium and water diuresis. However, if there is a pathophysiologic disruption in aldosterone, so that excessive amounts are present, both sodium and water retention will occur. Although there is a net increase in total body sodium, the ECF osmolarity is usually preserved, but, of course, there is great volume expansion of this compartment, since water will be reabsorbed through the tubules in an osmotic manner, to dilute the sodium that is reabsorbed. One example of such volume expansion is Cushing's syndrome, which is associated with hypersecretion of the adrenal cortex. The corticosteroids secreted in excessive amounts are thought to increase sodium reabsorption and to increase K^+ and H^+ secretion into the distal tubule. The patient therefore retains large amounts of sodium and water, loses potassium, and becomes alkalotic as well. Although edema and expanded ECF are features of this syndrome, usually the plasma concentration of sodium is normal, but hypernatremia can occur. A parallel example might be the patient with heart failure, who inappropriately secretes aldosterone, which causes excessive sodium and water reabsorption. Although the causes and end results of the two conditions are, of course, vastly different, nevertheless, at the level of the renal tubule, the primary process is increased sodium and water reabsorption. The patient with congestive heart failure is not able to adequately handle the expansion of the ECF, since the problem is related to the inability of the failing heart to pump blood forward in adequate amounts to perfuse the tissues. The aldosterone response is therefore pathophysiologic, since it will cause ever-greater plasma volumes, thus perpetuating the failure of the heart. A much more complete discussion of the effects of heart failure on fluid and electrolyte dynamics is presented in Chapter 6.

Treatment. The treatment of hypernatremia is aimed at (1) correcting the fluid alterations and (2) restoring ECF, and thus ICF, sodium levels to normal. In many cases the correction of the hydration problem will also correct the sodium concentration problem. It is important to note that correction of hypernatremia should not be accomplished rapidly, since cerebral edema has been reported to occur when fluid balance is too quickly restored.

8

Potassium imbalance

Potassium's major role in the body is to serve as the intracellular cation and to function as the determinant of the resting membrane potential (RMP) in most cells. Many metabolic cellular reactions are also dependent on the concentration of potassium. The intracellular and extracellular concentrations of potassium must be carefully regulated to ensure the steady state. Potassium is regulated through the kidneys, although some is lost in the sweat and in gastrointestinal secretions. The source of potassium is dietary (100 mEq/24 hr), and the absorption of potassium through the gastrointestinal mucosa is very efficient. Recall that the compartmentalization of potassium is nearly the reverse of that of sodium; that is, the normal cellular concentration is 150 to 160 mEq/liter, and the ECF concentration is about 3.5 to 5.5 mEq/liter. Fig. 8-1 indicates this compartmentalization in greater detail. Potassium is of course a cation and is therefore associated with anions within the ICF. This association results in the generation of the cell membrane resting potential, as described in detail in Chapter 3. Briefly, it is due to potassium diffusion through the cell membrane into the ECF that negative charges line up along the inner membrane surface, giving the inner membrane an electronegative polarity with regard to the outside surface. The negative anions that attempt to follow the potassium efflux are trapped by the impermeable membrane and cannot move through the membrane as well as can the easily diffusible potassium. Since potassium is the cell's most permeable ion, its diffusion accounts for most of the RMP. In fact, as the ratio of potassium in the ECF to potassium in the ICF increases, the RMP becomes proportionately more and more positive, and the membrane actually depolarizes because of the decreased net efflux of potassium, which occurs as a result of lessening of the diffusion gradient. The reverse is true when the ratio decreases, since more potassium diffuses out, more negativity lines up along the membrane, and the cell becomes

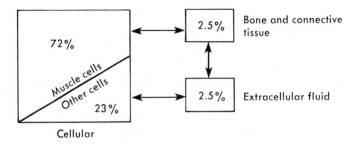

Fig. 8-1. Body potassium compartments.

hyperpolarized. The graph in Fig. 3-3 indicates these effects on RMP. Many of the signs and symptoms of potassium imbalance are therefore related to the effects of the RMP and cellular excitability.

Renal regulation of potassium balance is usually well controlled and keeps the extracellular potassium concentration within a tight range. It is also important to realize that whenever the ECF potassium concentration changes, there is often an equally likely alteration in the ICF potassium concentration. Cells can, in a sense, regulate the ECF potassium levels by increasing net efflux in potassium deficiency or increasing net influx in potassium excess. Both of these compensatory responses will change the potassium concentration of the cells as well as the ECF. However, the RMP is determined by the Nernst equation (p. 49), and therefore as long as the *ratio* of potassium inside and outside the cells is maintained, the RMP will not be affected. In significant hypokalemia or hyperkalemia this ratio is usually disturbed, and the cellular excitability is also changed through effects on the RMP.

Normally potassium is filtered by the kidneys at a concentration that is the same as in plasma, and all the potassium present in the glomerular filtrate is reabsorbed in the proximal convoluted tubule (PCT). In the distal convoluted tubule (DCT) and collecting ducts there is a variable secretion of potassium into the filtrate, depending on the body potassium stores and intracellular concentration. Cells rapidly take up any excess potassium that might be ingested in the diet and remove it from the ECF, where small rises may be significant in terms of the RMP. For example, a rise of 1 mEq/liter of potassium in the ECF represents close to a 20% rise in ECF potassium concentration, whereas the same rise in concentration in the ICF is a change of only 0.0067%. Thus the ECF concentration is usually maintained by the cellular uptake of ingested potassium or cellular release of potassium when the ECF concentration drops. The renal tubule cells contain 150 to 160 mEq/liter of potassium, as do other cells. Furthermore, they are highly permeable to potassium and will, in the presence of a concentration gradient, have increased diffusion of potassium out of the cell and into the tubular filtrate in the DCT. The concentration gradient is great because nearly all of the potassium initially present in the filtrate is reabsorbed in the PCT. Furthermore, this is enhanced by the flow rate of fluid moving through the DCT and collecting ducts. Since fluid moves quickly, the potassium present in the filtrate is rapidly washed through the tubule, and increasing amounts of potassium can diffuse out of the luminal cells and down the concentration gradient. For this reason potassium loss can occur when the urine flow rate is rapid, as in patients with osmotic diuresis (which is seen in diabetes mellitus, for example) or in patients treated with certain diuretics (furosemide [Lasix], chlorothiazide [Diuril], ethacrynic acid, mercurials). Potassium loss is also governed by the hormone aldosterone, which is directly regulated in a feedback manner by the serum levels of potassium. Hyperkalemia is a direct stimulus on the adrenal cortex. The mechanism of action of aldosterone is to increase K^+ and H^+ excretion. There is a relationship between sodium reabsorption by aldosterone and K^+ or H^+ secretion in distal tubular and collecting duct cells, but exactly what this relationship is and how the link occurs are unknown. There may be a relationship to linked pumping at the peritubular membrane, which involves an active transport carrier–mediated mechanism. In this model, sodium is pumped out of the cell (i.e., reabsorbed), and K^+ or H^+ is pumped in. These ions then diffuse down the electrical and concentration gradients into the tubular filtrate. There is considerable controversy over the model because the proportions of sodium reabsorbed to potassium secreted do not indicate linked pumping. One aspect of the model is that K^+ and H^+ compete for transport sites on the carrier system, and when K^+ concentration is high, there is a greater probability that K^+, rather than H^+, would occupy the sites. Of course, the result would be removal of potassium from the ECF, which is a desired effect in hyperkalemia, but the H^+ concentration of the ECF would also increase, causing metabolic acidosis. Exactly the reverse situation occurs when a primary increase in H^+ in the ECF or a drop in K^+ occurs. There is more transport of hydrogen, compared to potassium. In addition, in the first case hyperkalemia occurs, and in the second alkalosis occurs. The relationship of pH to serum potassium is indicated in Fig. 8-2.

That aldosterone is critical to normal potassium homeostasis is ap-

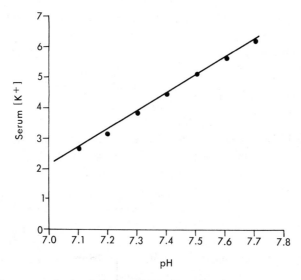

Fig. 8-2. Direct correlation between ECF pH and serum concentrations of K^+.

parent by the symptoms that develop in hypoadrenalism (e.g., Addison's disease). Hyperkalemia and resultant metabolic acidosis and cardiac changes are prominent features of this disease. In Cushing's syndrome, in which excessive corticosteroids are produced, there is hypokalemia and alkalosis.

PATHOPHYSIOLOGIC STATES
Hypokalemia

Hypokalemia is a state in which the ECF concentration of K^+ drops below 3.5 mEq/liter. This concentration is measured by determination of the serum electrolytes, which reflect the concentration of electrolytes throughout the ECF. Hypokalemia is a serious disturbance that may result in hyperpolarization of excitable cells and that has major effects on cardiac conduction and function. There is little tolerance for fluctuations in the ECF concentration of K^+, and normally any increases or decreases are quickly adjusted through cellular uptake or release and through renal mechanisms just described.

Causes of hypokalemia. The major causes of hypokalemia are as follows:

1. Use of diuretics
2. Diarrhea, vomiting, or other gastrointestinal losses
3. Alkalosis

4. Cushing's syndrome or adrenal hormone–producing tumors
5. Renal disease
6. Extreme diaphoresis

Hypokalemia may also be seen in patients recovering from burns, crush injuries, or massive trauma. Initially the ECF becomes hyperkalemic in these patients because of the release of potassium from damaged or dead cells, but this excess ECF concentration of potassium is excreted through the kidneys. When the patient begins to recover and becomes well hydrated, this potassium moves back from the ECF into the cells, and a state of hypokalemia can develop rather quickly. All the conditions that may result in hypokalemia will be further aided in their effect if the patient is not ingesting enough potassium in the diet. This fairly uncommon occurrence will rarely produce hypokalemia alone but may contribute to the problem if it already exists. Patients with hypokalemia are encouraged to eat foods high in potassium, including milk, orange juice, bananas, chocolate, meat, and many vegetables.

Influence of hypokalemia on excitability. Review of the Nernst equation (p. 49) indicates that a decrease in the ECF concentration of K^+, when it develops so rapidly that cellular K^+ concentration does not change, will cause the RMP to become more negatively charged on the inner surface, or hyperpolarized. Assuming that the cells' firing threshold is not altered, one can expect the cells to become less irritable and thus to require more stimulation strength over a longer period to fire. This, then, accounts for muscle weakness, fatigue, decreased strength, and behavioral changes that may take place in hypokalemia. It is of course possible that the *cellular* K^+ concentration would change in hypokalemia, particularly if the onset of the decrease is fairly slow. The cells would have a great diffusion gradient for passive potassium efflux, and this release of potassium into the ECF may result in a return of the ratio of K^+_{ICF} to K^+_{ECF} back to its normal value. Thus the RMP, according to the Nernst equation, is not affected. When the hypokalemia is chronic, the neuromuscular effects are therefore not as profound as in acute hypokalemia and hyperkalemia, in which the Nernst equation ratio is disturbed from normal.

Symptoms. The symptoms of hypokalemia depend on the rapidity of onset and individual differences. Symptoms related to the hyperpolarization of the cell membrane include sometimes profound muscle weakness, which affects both skeletal and smooth muscle. Nervous cells are also affected, and a decrease in irritability and conduction occurs. The effects are usually not severe, however, and may manifest themselves only

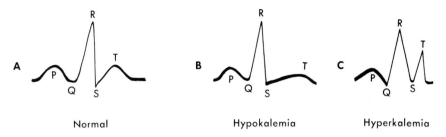

Fig. 8-3. **A,** Normal ECG. **B,** ECG of patient with hypokalemia. **C,** ECG of patient with hyperkalemia.

as mild confusion or lethargy. In nearly all hypokalemic patients with serum potassium values of less than 3 mEq/liter, cardiac conduction is altered very significantly. The electrocardiogram (ECG) changes are typical and include a depressed ST segment and a flattening of the T wave. The QRS complex may also become prolonged (Fig. 8-3). The myocardium responds to these significant abnormalities in conduction in various ways, including arrhythmias, bradycardia, and second-degree atrioventricular block. The presence of arrhythmias is further perpetuated in individuals receiving digitalis or diuretics or both. Hypokalemia increases the possibility of digitalis toxicity, and diuretics may cause potassium loss in the urine and thus promote hypokalemia. Other symptoms of hypokalemia relate to the effects on smooth muscle. Hypotonia of the gastrointestinal tract will lead to decreased motility, and as a result paralytic ileus may develop. Many patients with hypokalemia have polyuria and resultant polydypsia, which may be sequelae of renal tubule refractoriness to antidiuretic hormone (ADH). Apparently the action of ADH requires an adequate extracellular concentration of potassium. Since catecholamine refractoriness also occurs in hypokalemia, blood pressure regulation may be disturbed or, occasionally, postural hypotension or dizziness may occur. Table 8-1 indicates the contrasting methods of providing physical assessment for patients with hypokalemia and for those with hyperkalemia.

   Treatment. Treatment of hypokalemia is directed toward the underlying cause, if possible, and toward replacement of the potassium stores. Oral potassium is administered when the patient is able to tolerate oral fluids. Potassium chloride (KCl) is otherwise administered intravenously. Determination of the total amount of repair potassium needed is difficult. Potassium should not be administered at a concentration of greater than 40 mEq/liter, since it is an irritating substance and can cause local

Table 8-1. Physical assessment of potassium imbalance

	Cardiac system	Respiratory system	Neuromuscular system	Gastrointestinal system	Renal system
Hypokalemia					
Inspection		Increased work of breathing because of muscle weakness	Muscle weakness, cramps Confusion, lethargy "Flabby" muscles (especially leg muscles)	Anorexia Constipation	Polyuria
Palpation	Weak peripheral pulses			Distention	Mild peripheral edema
Percussion		Decreased diaphragmatic excursion Respirations shallow	↓ Deep tendon reflexes		
Auscultation	Tachycardia or bradycardia Arrhythmias Hypotension			↓ Bowel sounds	
Hyperkalemia					
Inspection			Irritability Muscle weakness Twitches	Diarrhea	Oliguria
Palpation			↓ Sensation, ↓ Point discrimination Paresthesias	Cramps	
Percussion			↑ Deep tendon reflexes ↑ Bowel sounds		
Auscultation	Bradycardia Arrhythmias				

tissue necrosis at the IV site. The rate of infusion should never exceed 20 mEq/hr. Usually the repair of the potassium deficit is done over several days, and the adequacy of the repair can be determined only by frequent measurement of the serum electrolytes. Approximately 400 mEq of potassium is required to increase the ECF potassium concentration by 1 mEq/liter in the hypokalemic patient. An important point to note is that potassium should never be administered to a patient until the adequacy of renal function is assured by good urinary output. Renal losses of potassium amount to about 50 mEq/24 hr, and if this loss suddenly ceases, there is a possibility that hyperkalemia will develop quickly and to a dangerous level, which may result in cardiac standstill.

Hyperkalemia

Hyperkalemia is a state in which the extracellular potassium concentration rises to a value greater than 5.5 mEq/liter. The same considerations that we have discussed for hypokalemia also hold true for hyperkalemia with regard to the effects of the potassium excess on the Nernst equation. If there is no great change in intracellular K^+ concentration, then hyperkalemia results in a drop in the RMP, or partial depolarization of excitable cells. Most of the symptoms associated with hyperkalemia are related to the effects on nerve, muscle, and the heart. When there is a rapid rise in potassium levels the effects develop quickly and are dramatic, particularly with regard to aberrations in cardiac conduction. If the rise in ECF potassium concentration is slower, there may be less effect on the RMP because some of the excess potassium in the ECF, as compared to that in the ICF, may return to nearly normal ratios. Furthermore, when hyperkalemia is severe, the RMP is initially depolarized and the cells become more excitable, but as the RMP rises to values close to and then beyond the threshold potential, the cells become less excitable. Therefore, early in the development of hyperkalemia, there may be signs of enhanced cellular irritability, but as the condition develops further the excitability of the cells diminishes. The cells, in other words, are at a resting potential in the refractory range, and they reach a point where they cannot respond to stimuli of any strength. With regard to the heart, this point results in cardiac standstill. The heart is the organ most sensitive to potassium excess, and of course problems in cardiac function are the most serious. Initially the heart is more excitable, with the sinoatrial (SA) node being the least sensitive and the atrioventricular node being the most sensitive to the effects of hyperkalemia. Therefore the SA node continues to discharge at close to the normal rate, but conduction is slower and the impulse may be blocked at the atrioventricular (AV) node. At high values of ECF potassium concentration the atria may dissociate from the ventricles, with ventricular fibrillation preceding the ultimate development of cardiac standstill in diastole. The ECG shows certain changes in hyperkalemia (Fig. 8-3). Notice that there is a widening of the QRS complex, peaked T waves, and prolongation of the PR segment.

Causes of hyperkalemia. The major causes of extracellular potassium excess, the most common being that associated with renal failure, are as follows:

1. Renal failure
2. Hypertonic dehydration
3. Massive cellular damage
4. Iatrogenic administration of large amounts of potassium intravenously
5. Hypoadrenalism (Addison's disease)
6. Acidosis

Whenever renal function is impaired and inadequate amounts of potassium are excreted, any other condition that may also result in hyperkalemia will be even more disturbing. Burned patients, for example, release large amounts of potassium into the ECF from the damaged, carbonized cells. Furthermore, there is usually a very great stress response in the burned patient, and intense vasoconstriction to preserve vascular volume is common. This will cause renal vasoconstriction and hypoxia, and renal failure may result if necrosis of the tubules occurs. Thus both the burn itself and the compensatory responses to it will contribute to the common development of hyperkalemia in these patients.

Symptoms. The symptoms of hyperkalemia are difficult to assess, and they vary among individuals. The most characteristic effect is on the ECG, and therefore when this diagnosis is expected or confirmed, the ECG should be very closely monitored. Other symptoms relate to the effects on neuromuscular function and smooth muscle hyperactivity. These changes are indicated in the assessment guide in Table 8-1.

Treatment. The treatment of hyperkalemia is directed at the cause, if possible, but since hyperkalemia can be such a life-threatening condition, the usual approach is to reduce the excessive ECF potassium value toward a more normal range. There are several approaches to this goal. One is to administer 10 ml of 10% calcium gluconate over several minutes intravenously for patients with severe hyperkalemia and cardiac involvement. Calcium acts on the threshold potential, whereas potassium alters the RMP. The cellular excitability can be restored toward normal in hyperkalemia by the calcium's action to lower the threshold potential (i.e., to make it more positive). This will allow depolarization and action potentials to develop and may restore normal cardiac conduction. Another common approach is to administer glucose and insulin, since insulin-induced transport into cells will be accompanied by entry of K^+ into the cells as well. Potassium can also be removed by dialysis in patients in renal failure. In addition, there are several preparations that bind potassium, including oral and enema preparations. Since these cation exchange resins bind potassium and relinquish sodium, they therefore will decrease the extracellular concentration of potassium and replace it with sodium.

Nurses caring for patients with hyperkalemia must be alert to the physiologic effects of excess potassium, continually assessing the patient and realizing that such a patient's status may change quickly and with little warning.

CASE STUDY • WOMAN WITH DIGITALIS TOXICITY

This case study represents a clinical situation that is often observed: digitalis toxicity as a sequela of hypokalemia. In this study the client developed diarrhea, which resulted in hypokalemia. The patient experienced arrhythmias and left-sided heart failure, which caused her to develop pulmonary edema. Many patients on digitalis preparations also receive diuretic therapy, which can result in potassium wasting. Such patients are particularly at risk for hypokalemia and digitalis intoxication during stresses such as physical illness.

HISTORY

Mrs. A. W., a 68-year-old widow and mother of four, had been living in the household of her eldest daughter since her husband's death 3 years ago. She had a history of diabetes, latent onset, which she controlled by dietary regimen and a daily dose of neutral protamine Hagedorn (NPH) insulin. In 1970 she experienced an anterior-wall myocardial infarction, and in 1975 the damage was extended to the lateral wall with a residual right bundle branch block. Since this time she had been seen on two separate occasions as a result of recurrent congestive heart failure. She was managed at home on digoxin (Lanoxin), 0.25 mg daily, and KCl elixir, 20 mEq daily.

PRESENT ILLNESS

She was brought to the emergency room on this admission by her daughter. Both the patient and her daughter attested to the fact that Mrs. W. had made strict efforts at controlling her weight and her sodium intake. They further related that her medical regimen has been followed as closely. Her latest symptoms began approximately 1 week before admission with an apparent intestinal virus and resultant diarrhea of 2 days' duration. Although the diarrhea had ceased now, she had been experiencing palpitations, shortness of breath, dizziness, and weakness. She denied chest pain but was orthopneic.

Physical examination by the emergency room nurse revealed an apprehensive client in moderate respiratory distress. The pulse rate was 64 beats/min and was weak and grossly irregular. The respiratory rate was 40/min, with rales and rhonchi heard bilaterally to both upper and lower lobes. Expiratory wheezes were heard throughout. Heart tones were distant, and blood pressure was 104/70 and faint. There was 1+ pedal edema bilaterally with moderate neck vein distention. The liver was somewhat enlarged but nontender. Bowel sounds were audible but hypoactive.

Since Mrs. W. was unable to tolerate a mask, oxygen was administered by nasal cannula at 4 liters/min. Her physician was notified of her arrival at the emergency room and advised of her condition. The following orders were then left:

> Admit to CCU: start IV fluids, 5% dextrose in water at TKO (to
>   keep open) rate
> Diagnosis: possible digitalis intoxication
> Serum electrolytes: stat
> Portable chest x-ray examination: stat
> ECG: stat
> Arterial blood gases: stat
> Digitalis level: stat
> Morphine sulfate: 4 mg IV push, 8 mg IM now
> Other orders to follow

After receiving morphine the client was then transferred to the coronary care unit (CCU). Arriving in the CCU, she was less apprehensive and less dyspneic although still experiencing some shortness of breath. She was oriented to the surroundings by the nurse, and her daughter was allowed to visit briefly. Her blood pressure remained stable at 110/70. Her respiratory rate was 32/min with mild effort. She had frequent coughing, productive of white, frothy sputum. There was no hemoptysis. Monitoring electrodes were attached to her chest wall for bedside cardiac monitoring, which revealed atrial fibrillation with a ventricular response of 58, including frequent ectopic beats.

The physician arrived shortly afterward to examine Mrs. W. and to review the laboratory work ordered in the emergency room. Serum electrolyte determinations revealed the following: sodium, 137; potassium, 3.0; chlorides, 97; calcium, 9.3. The arterial blood gas report was as follows: pH, 7.43; Pco_2, 46; Po_2, 80; saturation, 94% with a delta base of +3. The digitalis level was 2.8 ng. The ECG showed the right bundle block as before, although there was now a left axis deviation, suggesting left anterior hemiblock in addition. The ST segment was depressed, and low T waves were noted. The portable chest x-ray film showed left ventricular hypertrophy with a diffuse infiltrate throughout both fields, suggesting congestive heart failure of moderate degree.

After her old charts were reviewed and the current laboratory data analyzed, the physician left additional orders, including the following:

> KCl: 40 mEq/dl D_5W over 2 hr × 2 doses
> Spironolactone (Aldactone): 100 mg po, now and q6h
> KCl: 40 mEq po, now and q6h × 6 doses
> Repeat electrolytes in A.M.
> Insert Foley catheter: hourly outputs
> Phenytoin (Dilantin): 100 mg IV, now and q8h × 6 doses
> NPH insulin: 25 U subcu q A.M.
> Daily FBS
> 1000 kcal ADA diet with 1 gm sodium restriction
> Bed rest, with beside commode
> Nasal O_2: 3 to 5 liters/min prn
> Chloral hydrate (Noctec): 0.5 gm po at hs

A nursing care plan, drafted by the admitting nurse in the CCU, identified the following objectives as primary concerns:
1. Monitor cardiac rhythm closely until normal rate and rhythm are restored.
2. Monitor circulatory status closely until pulmonary and peripheral edema is resolved.
3. Monitor respiratory status closely until pulmonary edema is resolved and dyspnea alleviated.
4. Monitor diabetic state routinely unless unusual problems develop.

A long-range objective involved returning Mrs. W. to resumption of an activity level that would allow moderate housework and general self-care with minimal fatigue and an absence of dyspnea. Teaching measures would involve review of diet and activity alterations, as well as further instruction regarding her use of digitalis and diuretic therapy.

On the first night of her CCU admission, Mrs. W. was able to rest fairly comfortably, although the head of her bed remained elevated at least 30 degrees at her request. As a result of the diuretic therapy she produced 1600 ml of urine in an 8-hour period, with a continued good response from the spironolactone. Along with the increase in urinary output came subsequent relief of dyspnea. On the following morning she still exhibited rales, but these were confined to the bases. Her pedal edema had subsided as well. Her cardiac rhythm remained that of atrial fibrillation, although the ectopic activity had diminished greatly. Her serum potassium concentration had risen to 4.3 mEq/liter, and the order for oral KCl was reduced to only once daily. The oxygen was discontinued at the patient's request.

By the second morning after admission Mrs. W. was much improved. She was allowed to provide most of her personal care and could be out of bed and seated in a chair as she wished. She was subsequently transferred to the cardiac rehabilitation unit for further observation of her atrial fibrillation.

9

Calcium and phosphate imbalance

Calcium is a ubiquitous ion that plays important roles in membrane integrity and structure, electrophysiology, coagulation, and mechanical phenomena. Its plasma concentration is carefully regulated by several hormonal control mechanisms, a balance further maintained through the interaction of several body systems. The amount of absorbed and excreted calcium is under the primary control of the parathyroid gland, but this control requires the aid of vitamin D and depends on other ions' concentrations and gradients, which will be described later. The demand of various body tissues for calcium is another variable in this ion's homeostasis, since there are fluctuations in the body's need for calcium, depending, for example, on growth, bone stresses and remodeling, enzymatic demands, neurotransmission, the presence of fetal tissue, or disease. This discussion of calcium physiology will begin with a description of the normal distribution and role of calcium in various body systems. A discussion of calcium ion regulation and pathophysiologic mechanisms of calcium imbalance will follow, and general assessment strategies for any client with calcium imbalance with then be presented. The case study will point out the manifestations of calcium imbalance in one particular client.

DISTRIBUTION OF CALCIUM

Calcium, an alkaline earth-metal cation, is present in three chemical forms in the body fluids: (1) ionized (4.5 mg/dl), (2) nondiffusible, which is calcium complexed to protein anions (5 mg/dl), and (3) calcium salts such as calcium citrate and calcium phosphate (1 mg/dl). These forms of calcium constitute a relatively small fraction of the total body calcium, however. The great proportion of calcium is found in bones and teeth in the form of inert hydroxyapatite crystals. In terms of physiologic activity it is the ionized form of calcium (Ca^{++}) that is active, and an equilibrium exists between the complexed forms and the free ion in the body fluids:

$$Ca\text{-protein} + H^+ \rightleftarrows Ca^{++} + H\text{-protein}$$

Thus the state of calcium is influenced by the pH; a drop in pH favors the formation of nondiffusible calcium-protein complexes, as well as calcium salts. This result is due to the law of mass action, which states that the speed of a reaction is proportional to the concentrations of the products and reactants. Since the above equation is a reversible reaction, a drop in the concentration of one of the reactants will result in a driving of the reaction toward the formation of that reactant. In the case of a drop in H^+, which changes the pH of the system toward a more alkaline state, the effect on the reaction will be toward the formation of H^+, which can be accomplished only by slowing the forward reaction and increasing the speed of the reverse reaction. This effect will, however, decrease the ionized calcium concentration and increase the concentration of the complexed calcium. The reverse would of course take place if the H^+ should increase, with a driving of the reaction toward the right and a resultant increase in the Ca^{++} concentration. Both of these effects are seen clinically in patients with either alkalosis or acidosis. In alkalosis, for example, a drop in the serum concentration of Ca^{++} may occur, resulting in a state of hypocalcemia, which may give rise to actual signs of tetany. This pH effect on the equilibrium has been regarded as important physiologically. There is recent evidence, however, that the Ca^{++} imbalances that occur in altered pH states are not the result of an effect on chemical equilibria but rather are due to other direct Ca^{++}-H^+ interactions, perhaps on the cellular level.

Calcium's concentration in the ECF is regulated chiefly through the parathyroid and thyroid glands. The balance among bone calcium release or uptake, gut absorption, and kidney excretion is determined by parathyroid hormone (PTH) and thyrocalcitonin, although several other hormones (e.g., growth hormone, cortisone) do influence calcium balance to some degree. Of the total body calcium, 99% is present in bone in two major compartments. These are the exchangeable and nonexchangeable calcium compartments, the former being in equilibrium with the ECF calcium. Bone is a highly active tissue that is constantly being remodeled even during adult life. The yearly turnover of calcium is nearly 20% of the total bone calcium. Bone remodeling requires breakdown of the crystalline structure of the bone, with release of the minerals, and then rebuilding to accommodate the new stresses placed on the bone.

Formation of bone

To understand the regulation of calcium in the body fluids, one must appreciate the mechanisms of bone formation and breakdown. The reason is that these processes are regulated by PTH and thyrocalcitonin to some degree and are therefore intrinsic to the maintenance of the normal serum concentration of calcium.

Bone is a connective tissue containing several types of bone cells (osteoblasts, osteocytes, and osteoclasts), a matrix of collagen and other fibers, and a mineral that is deposited in a specific pattern on the collagen. The hydroxyapatite crystal $(Ca_{10}[PO_4]_6[OH]_2)$ is the major mineral. Other mineral forms of calcium phosphate are present, however, and other bone-seeking chemicals may also be present (e.g., fluoride, strontium, lead). There are two mechanisms of bone formation: intramembranous ossification and cartilage replacement. The first takes place in flat bones such as the skull and involves the formation of layers of bone by osteoblasts on a matrix of connnective tissue membrane. The second is the mechanism of long bone growth and takes place at the epiphyses, which are plates of cartilage located at the ends of long bones. As the bone grows, the cartilage in the epiphyseal plate becomes replaced by bone. Active epiphyses are present throughout childhood and become closed, or fully ossified, only when all growth has ceased.

Bone contains a canalicular system by which the osteocytes, which are the mature bone cells, communicate and are nourished. There is evidence that osteocytes may be responsive to PTH and can participate in bone breakdown (resorption) by releasing enzymes that aid in the release of Ca^{++} from the hydroxyapatite crystal. Osteoblasts are primitive bone-forming cells, and it is likely that they become transformed into osteocytes and become embedded in the bone that they participate in forming. Osteoblasts are usually located at the surface of growing bone.

For bone to be formed properly so that it is best able to function in support of the body weight, it must constantly be remodeled even as it forms. Osteoclasts play the major role in the process. Osteoclasts are giant, multinucleated cells that are intensely mobile, phagocytic, and secretory. They secrete a variety of enzymes that are osteolytic, breaking down the mineral of bone and releasing Ca^{++} and phosphate. Osteoclasts are also sensitive to PTH, but their responsiveness is much slower than that of the osteocytes.

Bone formation therefore requires osteoblasts to lay down the bone and osteoclasts to model the bone as it grows. Furthermore, osteoclasts play a major role in bone remodeling in the adult, in which actual bone growth has ceased. In the adult, when stresses on bone change, the osteoclasts are stimulated to destroy the old bone and thus allow osteoblasts to form the bone tissue in a new functional arrangement.

Bone resorption. Bone resorption is stimulated by PTH when the serum concentration of calcium drops. The resultant breakdown of the mineral releases calcium from the bone, and this calcium then exchanges with the plasma quite freely so that serum levels of calcium will increase as the result of PTH-stimulated bone resorption. The action of PTH is very rapid, with effects on resorption occurring within minutes. The calcium that is exchangeable with ECF is therefore believed to be responsive to PTH and may consist of several different sources of calcium. There may be some surface calcium that is readily exchangeable in this compartment, but it appears that the bulk of exchangeable calcium requires osteocytic breakdown of the mineral. The actual mechanism by which PTH stimulates osteocytes to resorb bone is under investigation in many laboratories. Long-term effects of PTH, in states of chronic hypocalcemia, for example, may affect bone accretion more strongly, causing both less formation and increased resorption. The net effects over time are a leeching out of calcium from bone, a loss of bone mass, and a tendency for the bone to weaken and more easily fracture.

ROLE OF CALCIUM

Calcium plays a major role in cell membrane–related phenomena. For example, it maintains membrane gradients for certain ions, stabilizes the membrane phospholipids for structural integrity, and acts as a cofactor in several important membrane enzyme functions. Calcium is considered a necessary component of the cell membrane, and interruption of the normal membrane calcium concentration has profound effects on membrane structure and functions. The amount of calcium present, however, is incredibly small. We think of calcium as imparting stiffness or rigidity to the membrane and therefore its absence as allowing greater flexibility and fluidity. Since the cell membrane is like an oily fluid, it appears that the appropriate calcium concentration within the membrane gives this membrane oil enough stiffness to impart actual structure. The cell membrane is extremely impermeable to extracellular calcium and actively pumps out excess calcium that does leak in. Membrane calcium is probably chelated by phospholipids within the membrane at their polar head groups. It is speculated that as cells age they accumulate more Ca^{++} as both their transport efficiency declines and the number of molecules available to chelate calcium decreases. Senescent erythrocytes, for example, are more rigid, less deformable, and ultimately more fragile than young erythrocytes and therefore are subject to hemolysis and phagocytosis in the spleen. As the membrane concentration of calcium increases, there are deleterious effects on membrane protein as well. This is most dramatically demonstrated by the transformation of normal erythrocytes into sea urchin–shaped cells (echinocytes) when red cells are incubated in a medium containing a large amount of calcium. Perhaps calcium is echinocytogenic in that it causes abnormal conformation of membrane protein, which in turn results in protein contraction and spicule development on the membrane surface.

Membrane calcium, through its interaction with both phospholipid and protein, affects the structure of the membrane. Furthermore, there is a role for calcium in membrane permeability. It is believed that calcium stabilizes the membrane in a manner that *opposes* sodium transport. One theory is that Ca^{++} competes with Na^{++} for cell membrane receptor sites. Therefore an excess of calcium acts to saturate more binding sites than normal, causing less sodium to bind, and thus less sodium is able to enter the cell. The opposite occurs when decreased amounts of calcium are present in the ECF and when larger amounts of sodium move across the membrane. Thus cellular excitability is influenced in states of hypercalcemia or hypocalcemia because sodium diffusion is the mechanism whereby cells reach threshold and fire action potentials. An excess of calcium decreases cellular excitability by raising the threshold for firing, whereas a reduction in ECF concentrations of calcium causes greater excitability and subsequently a state of tetany, in which muscle cells are in a continuous state of excitation-contraction.

Calcium appears to play a part in membrane enzymatic action as well as in cell formation and permeability. There are at least two forms of membrane-bound adenosinetriphosphatase (ATPase) involved in active transport processes, one of which is activated by Mg^{++} and the other by Ca^{++}. The Ca^{++}-activated ATPase may be involved in the active transport of Ca^{++} out of the cell. The Mg^{++}-activated ATPase is the form responsible in part for active Na^+-K^+ transport. Calcium inhibits this latter form of ATPase and therefore inhibits the sodium pump. It is theoretically possible that the rate of pumping of Na^+ and K^+ is regulated by the amount of ionized calcium available in the microenvironment of the cell membrane. Calcium is also a candidate for coenzymatic function in several

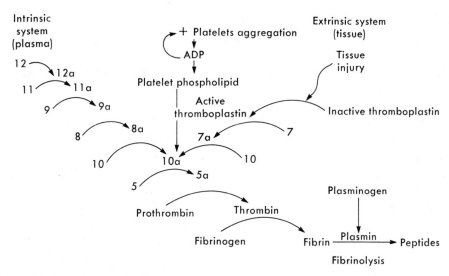

Fig. 9-1. Blood coagulation. Intrinsic and extrinsic systems of coagulation, in concert with effects of platelet aggregation, yield activated factors that produce a cascading effect, ultimately leading to formation of strands of fibrin. Fibrin is broken down through action of plasmin. (From Groër, M. E., and Shekleton, M. E.: Basic pathophysiology: a conceptual approach, St. Louis, 1979, The C. V. Mosby Co.)

other enzyme systems that are membrane bound. These systems include acetylcholine release and several different cellular exocytotic processes. To bind the appropriate chemicals, some cell receptors require Ca^{++}.

Aside from its important membrane functions, calcium phosphate is the major mineral of bones and teeth. The bone concentration of calcium also serves as a storage compartment for Ca^{++} and is a source of replenishment of plasma Ca^{++} when a balance cannot be maintained by either increased gut absorption or decreased kidney excretion. Exchangeable bone Ca^{++} is under the control of PTH and thyrocalcitonin, which operate through negative feedback loops to regulate plasma concentrations of Ca^{++}. Basically, PTH is released whenever the plasma concentration of Ca^{++} drops below the set point for the feedback loop and acts to increase bone Ca^{++} release. Thyrocalcitonin acts in states of hypercalcemia (>12 mg/dl) to cause increased uptake of Ca^{++} into the bone as one of its effects. These mechanisms will be described in greater detail shortly. Calcium functions in coagulation in several important ways, and its absence will inhibit the coagulation cascade (Fig. 9-1). One role of Ca^{++} is involved with platelet physiology. These corpuscles initiate the sealing of an injured surface and aggregate into increasingly larger masses. The Ca^{++} in intracellular platelets appears to be involved in this reaction, which is mediated through platelet membrane adenyl cyclase. The platelet plug that forms functions along with activated factor X and Ca^{++} to allow the enzymatic conversion of prothrombin to thrombin. Thrombin then participates in the conversion of fibrinogen to fibrin, which is the actual fibrous meshwork of a complete clot. The Ca^{++} also participates in the coagulation cascade—for example, in the conversion of inactive to active factor IX and in the formation of activated factor VIII (the antihemophilic factor). Although the absence of Ca^{++} in the test tube will inhibit the coagulation process, an analogous effect on coagulation in vivo is seldom, if ever, seen, since the degree of hypocalcemia required to produce coagulation problems is a Ca^{++} value of 2.5 mg/dl. This level of Ca^{++} is incompatible with life. Therefore it can be said that although Ca^{++} is an absolute requirement for coagulation, the assessment of coagulability in the hypocalcemic patient does not assume great importance.

Calcium functions in excitation-contraction in all forms of muscle. Its action in muscle was described briefly in Chapter 3.

Skeletal muscle

Recall that there are two systems of channels within muscle cells: the T system and the sarcoplasmic reticulum. The tubules of the T system are continuous with the external cell membrane and thus provide for the possibility of exchange between the external and internal environments of the muscle cell. The major role of the T system in muscle contraction is somewhat like that of an electrical wiring system. The electrical depolarization that results from the neuromuscular transmission across the myoneural synapse not only affects the muscle cell membrane (sarcolemma) but also is further perpetuated throughout the interior of the cell via the T system. The tubules of the T system penetrate deeply into the muscle cell and carry the wave of depolarization into the sarcomeric units of myofilaments, which then ultimately respond by sliding. However, as we have seen, contraction also requires Ca^{++}. The sarcoplasmic reticulum stores Ca^{++}, releasing it when the cell membrane and T system become excited. The T system and the sarcoplasmic reticulum actually cross over each other, and at the T band the tubules of both systems form an arrangement known as the *triad*. When the membrane excitation transmits through the T system, the sarcoplasmic reticulum releases stored Ca^{++}, which then initiates contraction. Agents that increase the movement of Ca^{++} into the cell also increase muscular contraction strength by increasing the binding of troponin C to Ca^{++} (Chapter 3).

Smooth muscle

Smooth muscle contraction also requires Ca^{++}, but many of the details of its action are not known. If Ca^{++} availability is somehow decreased in smooth muscle, the contractility of the muscle also decreases. It is believed that the mechanism of action of the sympathetic nervous system on the gastrointestinal tract is in part explained by effects on Ca^{++}. Norepinephrine is the neurotransmitter released by nerves of the sympathetic system, and its effects on the gastrointestinal tract are decreased motility and secretion through (1) increased binding of Ca^{++} inside cells and (2) increased diffusion of Ca^{++} out of cells. Both mechanisms would of course decrease the amount of Ca^{++} available to initiate contraction.

Cardiac muscle

Calcium's function in cardiac contractility is a subject of much research. It appears that Ca^{++} participates electrically in the action potential, as well as in the mechanics of muscle contraction. Since cardiac problems are a major sign of calcium concentration changes, the function of Ca^{++} in heart physiology will be explored in some detail.

The cardiac muscle cell differs from the skeletal muscle cell in several important ways. The functions of both require Ca^{++}, but the skeletal muscle cell is not closely dependent on an adequate supply of extracellular Ca^{++}. The Ca^{++} used in excitation-contraction is available intracellularly, and the sarcoplasmic reticulum is a Ca^{++} compartment that does not require continuous Ca^{++} input from the ECF for every contraction in order to maintain the appropriate Ca^{++} concentration within it. (This does not imply, however, that changes in serum concentrations of Ca^{++} do not have eventual effects on skeletal muscle contraction.) Contrasted with the apparent independence of skeletal muscle on external Ca^{++} for internal Ca^{++} release, the mammalian heart muscle is dependent on external Ca^{++} on a beat-for-beat basis. Ca^{++} current actually moves into the heavy muscle cells with depolarization. However, there is a developed sarcoplasmic reticulum in heart muscle cells, and experiments have shown that it is capable of release and uptake of Ca^{++} in apparently the same manner as skeletal muscle. Fig. 9-2 diagrams a proposed model for Ca^{++} current in the adult mammalian ventricle. Here we see that Ca^{++} movement into the cell is coupled to Na^{+} efflux and that the Ca^{++} acts on the sarcoplasmic reticulum to stimulate it to release its stored Ca^{++} into the myofilaments. This figure illustrates the hypothesis of *Ca^{++}-induced release of Ca^{++}* from the sarcoplasmic reticulum. Although this theory has not been definitely accepted among all cardiac electrophysiologists, there are many who accept it in one form or another.

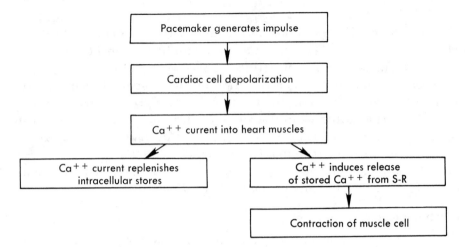

Fig. 9-2. Ca^{++} current is believed to occur as heart muscle cell is depolarized, perhaps as Na^+ is being pumped out. It may be responsible for plateau of action potential. Ca^{++} induces release of Ca^{++} stored in sarcoplasmic reticulum, and it also replenishes depleted Ca^{++} stores. Muscle cell contraction is the result.

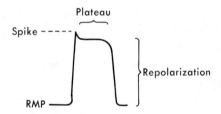

Fig. 9-3. Ventricular muscle cell action potential.

Calcium current has been suggested in the maintenance of the cardiac muscle cell's plateau (Fig. 9-3). It is seen that the initial spike in the ventricular muscle fiber is a rapid depolarization of the membrane after threshold is reached. This spike is followed by a plateau of approximately 150 msec, and then a rapid repolarization occurs. Inward Ca^{++} current as well as Na^+ current is thought to be responsible for the action potential's particular waveform in cardiac muscle cells. Certain drugs with cardiac actions appear to act on Ca^{++} availability, and altered states of serum calcium concentration can have serious effects on cardiac contractility.

CALCIUM AND PHOSPHATE RELATIONSHIP

The hydroxyapatite crystalline lattice of bone is made up of both Ca^{++} and phosphate. Phosphate is a buffer anion that is present both intracellularly and extracellularly. Phosphate concentration is regulated by PTH and by activated vitamin D. The normal serum value of phosphate ranges from 3 to 12 mg/dl. Phosphate is absorbed through the gastrointestinal mucosa, an action facilitated by vitamin D. Its precipitation as bone mineral and its renal excretion are also controlled by vitamin D and by PTH, as is calcium regulation.

The product of the concentrations of Ca^{++} and phosphate in the serum is a constant. Thus, if one ion changes, then the constant can be maintained only by an inverse fall or rise in the other ion. If hypercalcemia develops, the phosphate decreases and vice versa. This relationship must be maintained in the body so that the product of Ca^{++} and phosphate does not exceed the solubility product for the reaction ($Ca^{++} + HPO_4$). When this is exceeded, $CaHPO_4$ forms as a precipitate within many body tissues.

Furthermore, excessive $CaHPO_4$ formation depletes the body stores of ionized calcium, and hypocalcemia develops. This sequence of events is seen in renal failure, in which the kidneys are not able to excrete phosphate or form activated vitamin D. The excessive phosphate causes an inverse drop in Ca^{++} through the chemical equilibrium described above, and hypocalcemia results. Of course, hypocalcemia causes PTH release, which acts to stimulate phosphate excretion from the kidney, but if severe renal disease is present, this cannot be accomplished. The pathophysiologic events that occur result in bone disease such as osteitis fibrosa cystica and osteomalacia. The calcification of soft tissue also has profound pathophysiologic effects on many organ systems.

ACTION OF PARATHYROID HORMONE, THYROCALCITONIN, AND VITAMIN D
Parathyroid hormone

The parathyroid glands are four small bodies located in the neck just behind the thyroid gland. So difficult are they to distinguish from thyroid tissue that they are sometimes inadvertently removed during thyroidectomy. Their only known function is to secrete PTH, which is regulated through negative feedback by the blood calcium level. The hormone is a small polypeptide (molecular weight 8500) consisting of 84 amino acids. It is produced by the *chief* cells in the parathyroid gland. These cells appear remarkably sensitive to a drop in serum concentrations of calcium, responding by an appropriate output of the hormone. The action of the hormone is on three major target organs: bone, gastrointestinal mucosa, and the kidneys. It may possibly affect the lactating breast as well.

The PTH promotes *resorption* of bone, a process defined as bone breakdown to release calcium and phosphate. The hormone inhibits collagen synthesis, activates osteocytes, and stimulates the activity of osteoclasts.

The action of PTH on the gastrointestinal mucosa is controversial. Although some researchers believe that there is a direct effect, most argue for an indirect stimulation of Ca^{++} absorption through the mediation of vitamin D. The presence of PTH is required for the activation of vitamin D, and the active form of this vitamin is known to act on the intestinal epithelium. The amount of Ca^{++} taken in by diet is about 0.6 to 1.0 gm/24 hr in Americans. The maximum that can be transported daily through the gastrointestinal mucosa into the bloodstream is 300 mg, however. The mechanism of transport involves active transport into the small intestinal mucosal cells, followed by diffusion into the intestinal capillaries. Phosphate may be transported with Ca^{++}, although this is not clear. Activated vitamin D is an absolute requirement for Ca^{++} transport, although very small amounts are needed to produce a great effect. The vitamin is considered to act hormonally and produces its effect through changes in the cellular synthesis of ribonucleic acid (RNA). Synthesis of a transporting protein may theoretically be induced by the presence of vitamin D hormone. Another possible effect may be on a Ca^{++}-ATPase, which is necessary for Ca^{++} transport across the intestinal epithelium. It has further been observed that similar effects on both phosphate and amino acid transport in the gut are produced by vitamin D. Phosphate absorption differs, however, from Ca^{++} in that the amount absorbed depends on the dietary intake, and excesses are absorbed and then later excreted through the kidneys, whereas Ca^{++} transport is limited.

The action of PTH on the kidneys is of great importance for Ca^{++} regulation. Slightly more than half of the Ca^{++} in the plasma is actually filtered through the glomerulus, and about 70% of this filtrate is reabsorbed in the PCT. Further reabsorption occurs in the loop of Henle, and a small amount occurs in the DCT and collecting tubules. The action of PTH, which is to increase Ca^{++} reabsorption, appears to occur only in the latter two parts of the nephron. PTH-sensitive transport is *active* transport but involves a different mechanism from that of Na^+-K^+ transport. Some research has suggested that the mechanism of action of PTH is through activation of sensitive transporting cell adenyl cyclase. The intracellular formation of the second messenger, cyclic adenosine monophosphate (cAMP), would then be stimulated. This mechanism has not been demonstrated in the kidneys of all species, however. Possible actions of cAMP could be to increase the cell's permeability to Ca^{++}, to alter the cellular metabolism, or to stimulate the formation of transporting proteins by the sensitive renal cells.

Vitamin D

Vitamin D is both ingested in the diet and synthesized in the body and, through its hormonelike actions, is indispensable in the regulation of Ca^{++}. Vitamin D is actually the name given to a group of similar compounds that become activated in various body tissues. Cholecalciferol (vitamin D_3) is first produced in the skin from a provitamin precursor through the action of ultraviolet light. Vitamin D_3 is also included in most American diets. The essential nature of this first sunlight-requiring conversion is exemplified by the occurrence of rickets in English children during the industrial revolution. Factory-produced smog obscured the sunlight, and inadequately fed children began to lose Ca^{++} from their bones and to absorb little Ca^{++} through their gastrointestinal tract. The result was a softening and bending of the bones, which gave rise to characteristic skeletal anomalies. When these affected children were moved to the rural areas of England, they were often able to recover. However, rickets during childhood can result in irreversible bone changes and deformities.

Vitamin D_3 is not metabolically active but must be chemically changed in the liver to 25-hydroxycholecalciferol by a hydroxylation process. This compound is further metabolized in kidney tissue, a process that apparently requires PTH, and is stimulated by hypophosphatemia. The metabolite that the kidney tissue forms is 1,25-dihydroxycholecalciferol, and it is the most active form of vitamin D. Physiologically, it acts as a hormone by traveling through the bloodstream and acting on distant target organs. The general actions of vitamin D are to increase Ca^{++} uptake from the gastrointestinal tract and to participate with PTH in bone resorption.

Thyrocalcitonin

Thyrocalcitonin is an important hormone in Ca^{++} regulation when serum values rise to levels above 12 mg/dl. It is produced by the thyroid gland, but recent evidence indicates that it is also produced at other sites in the body; many physiologists therefore refer to it only as calcitonin. Thyrocalcitonin acts to inhibit bone resorption when the serum concentration of Ca^{++} increases to hypercalcemic levels. The mechanism of action is not known, but numerous theories suggest that inhibition of cAMP formation or inhibition of bone Ca^{++} release at the cellular level may be affected by thyrocalcitonin. The overall effect of the hormone is to lower serum concentrations of Ca^{++} and phosphate.

DIETARY SOURCES OF CALCIUM

The role, distribution, and regulation of Ca^{++} have been described. An important corollary to this information is a knowledge of food sources of Ca^{++}. One cause of hypocalcemia is inadequate intake of Ca^{++}, vitamin D, or protein. The latter is required in the diet so that adequate Ca^{++} will be available to cells. The reason is that low serum albumin will ultimately cause low Ca^{++}, since nearly half of the serum Ca^{++} is albumin bound. Calcium absorption in the gut is also dependent on the phosphorus present in the diet. If too much phosphorus is present, it will bind to Ca^{++} and precipitate in the gut as the solubility product is reached; therefore neither mineral will be absorbed. The optimal ratio of Ca^{++} to phosphorus in the normal, nonpregnant, nonlactating adult is 1:1.5. Many other anions commonly present in food will also bind Ca^{++}. High-protein diets, which are often also high in phosphate, will inhibit Ca^{++} absorption.

The major sources of Ca^{++} in the American diet are dairy products, whole or enriched grain foods, and leafy green vegetables. Vitamin D–fortified milk helps provide this vitamin in adequate quantities, but other food sources include butter, margarine, and egg yolks.

PATHOPHYSIOLOGIC ALTERATIONS IN CALCIUM BALANCE
Hypocalcemia

Recall that the normal serum calcium is in both ionized and bound forms, the ionized form being physiologically active. A state of hypocalcemia exists when the serum concentration of calcium drops below 8.5 mg/dl, which reflects a drop in ionized calcium to less than 4 mg/dl. This of course assumes that the plasma concentration of albumin, which binds Ca^{++}, does not drop.

Calcium deficit can develop in many different ways. Hypocalcemia might result if blood transfusions containing citrate are administered very rapidly, since citrate combines with Ca^{++} and essentially removes the ionized form from the blood. The development of hypocalcemia has been described in this chapter as the result of hyperphosphatemia. Another cause is hypoalbuminemia, which occurs in many types of pathophysiologic alterations. Examples of the latter include liver disease, starvation, and the nephrotic syndrome. Of course, parathyroid disease could lead to hypocalcemia as the result of decreased PTH output. Another common cause is vitamin D deficiency as the result of either poor diet or inadequate exposure to sunlight. This problem could also develop in a variety of gastrointestinal tract diseases in which fat-soluble vitamins are poorly absorbed. Inadvertent removal of the parathyroid glands during surgery is also one of the possible causes of hypocalcemia, as is the administration of certain drugs (ACTH, glucagon, EDTA). Several neoplastic processes result in metastatic invasion of the bone, which in turn inhibits bone resorption and appears also to increase calcium deposition into bone. Pancreatitis is associated with hypocalcemia because of the release of pancreatic lipase into the ECF and tissue, which causes lipolysis. The fatty acids formed combine with Ca^{++} to form Ca^{++} soaps, and this process results in a drop in ionized calcium. Another cause of hypocalcemia is pregnancy, since Ca^{++} requirements increase about 50% at this time, and mild hypocalcemia may develop if inadequate amounts are taken in the diet.

Hyperventilation should also be mentioned because it produces hypocalcemia through its pH effect.

Signs and symptoms. Many of the signs and symptoms of hypocalcemia can be predicted once an understanding of calcium physiology is attained. The important aspects of calcium's role in the body have been discussed in great detail so that the effects of hypocalcemia will be understandable. Since Ca^{++} plays such a major role in neuromuscular excitability, it is obvious that a drop in ionized calcium will produce symptoms in this area of function. Calcium deficit results in a partial depolarization of the nerve and muscle cell membranes. In particular, the threshold potential is increased, reaching a value that is closer to the membrane potential. Thus the membrane does not require much depolarization before it discharges an action potential.

Particular signs and symptoms of neuromuscular excitability include cramping of muscles, spasms, convulsions, mental confusion and even psychotic behavior, paresthesias of many different types but occurring particularly in the hands and feet and in and around the mouth, and ultimately the development of *tetany*. Tetany is the name given to a clinical syndrome of excessive continuous muscle contraction, laryngeal spasm and stridor, paresthesias, and carpopedal spasm (spasm of muscles in both hands and feet), which gives rise to a characteristic flexion and adduction (Fig. 9-4). Tetany can interfere with oxygenation as the indi-

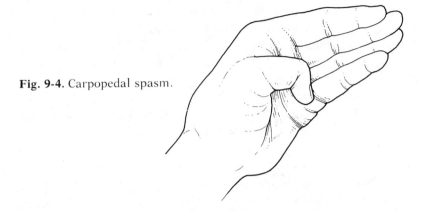

Fig. 9-4. Carpopedal spasm.

vidual struggles to breathe, and severe dyspnea can cause death. Another effect of hypocalcemia is on cardiac excitability. Most commonly, there may be prolongation of the Q-T interval on the ECG, which indicates a delay in ventricular depolarization and repolarization. This delay may become significant enough to result in heart failure, although this is not common. The cardiac muscle contractility is also affected, since a Ca^{++} current is required for every contraction, and hypocalcemia will result in less available Ca^{++} in the ECF for this mechanical event. The gastrointestinal tract will occasionally be affected in hypocalcemia, with resultant cramping and diarrhea.

Hypocalcemia may either develop acutely or occur more slowly. There are wide ranges of response to hypocalcemia, depending on the rapidity of onset and the presence of chronic hypocalcemia. Some persons with hypocalcemia of long standing have minimal or no symptoms, but chronic problems that do develop include fatigability, skin lesions, and emotional lability. Among the more common problems associated with chronic hypocalcemia are the development of cataracts and certain changes in hair, bones, nails, and teeth.

Physical assessment and treatment

History. Assessment of hypocalcemia involves an initial thorough history and inspection of the patient's affect, memory, and emotional state, as well as any alteration of previous normal behavior. Such changes may be subtle at first but eventually may progress to excessive irritability and unreasonableness. The history of therefore of great importance, and data related to any unusual sensations the patient has been experiencing should be collected. There is a wide range of descriptions given to scalp paresthesias, for example. The patient may feel a prickly sensation or may state that the hair feels as though it were standing on end. "Pins and needles" is the most common description that patients ascribe to paresthesias caused by hypocalcemia. The patient may, however, have difficulty speaking, and then the history is usually obtained from relatives or friends.

Neuromuscular assessment. Inspection of the neuromuscular function is of the greatest importance, since most of the symptoms of hypocalcemia arise from excessive irritability. Tics, fasciculations, and spasms may all be present. They are often repetitive and are particularly aggravated by external sensory stimuli. The act of swallowing may bring on an attack of laryngeal spasm, which will of course cause great anxiety. The patient may respond to a loud noise or a sudden bright light by a sudden string of muscular spasms. Obviously, such patients require a very quiet, stable environment while undergoing treatment.

Neuromuscular assessment also includes examination of the deep tendon reflexes (patellar, Achilles, biceps, and triceps) because these are usually hyperactive. Two useful signs of tetany are Chvostek's and Trousseau's signs. Chvostek's sign is a spasm of the facial muscles when the face is percussed just in front of the ear. Percussion of the facial nerve is a stimulus that will lead to spasm of muscles on one side of the face, sometimes including even the eyelids. Trousseau's sign is the production of ischemia-induced carpal spasm in the hypocalcemic patient by application of a tourniquet or blood pressure cuff on the forearm for at least 3 minutes. It should be noted that occasionally completely normal individuals will have positive Chvostek's and Trousseau's signs, and on the other hand, they may be absent in some individuals who are hypocalcemic.

Chest assessment. Respiratory assessment assumes great importance in the patient with fully developed tetany, since the work of breathing is greatly increased and the attendant anxiety creates a vicious cycle whereby muscular contractions are even further enhanced. (It should also be kept in mind that an occasional client will develop hypocalcemia as the result of hyperventilation, most often as part of an anxiety reaction. Therefore, in a differentiation of the possible causes of tetany, respiratory assessment is necessary.) Furthermore, in the patient with tetany and rigor of the jaw, laryngeal spasms and involuntary and often painful spasms of the accessory muscles of respiration may lead to a variety of effects. Diminished breath sounds and adventitial sounds are likely to develop. If the patient also develops congestive heart failure, signs and symptoms of backward heart failure may be superimposed on the respiratory tract involvement. Careful auscultation of the chest is done to determine the degree of airway resistance, the relative amount of work required for breathing, the possible inadequacy of ventilation at the alveolar level, the possible presence of adventitial breath sounds and cardiac failure. Routine electrocardiography should be performed to determine whether altered conduction is present. The strength, rate, and quality of peripheral pulses must also be routinely assessed by palpation.

Gastrointestinal assessment. Bowel sounds may be hyperactive and abdominal cramping very severe in the patient with tetany. The pain may actually mimic that caused by an acute abdominal condition requiring surgery. Therefore the gastrointestinal system is carefully evaluated by inspection, auscultation, palpation, and percussion.

Treatment. The diagnosis of tetany dictates immediate treatment, since this condition is life threatening in its most severe form. After laboratory serum values show hypocalcemia, intravenous administration of calcium gluconate in a 10% solution is begun. As soon as the patient is able the replacement can be done orally, and careful monitoring of the serum concentrations of Ca^{++} will dictate the dosage of oral replacement. Of course, diagnosis of hypocalcemic tetany is not sufficient, since this condition is a sign of another disease process. Therefore a complete diagnostic study of parathyroid gland function and investigation of other etiologies of hypocalcemia are required after the patient is no longer acutely ill. The acute phase of the illness may require intensive nursing care, frequent monitoring of blood gases and respiratory and cardiovascular functioning, and ongoing assessment of the neurologic and muscular involvement. Seizure precautions should be routine, as well as the availability of an airway, a tracheostomy set, and a ventilator. Bronchodilating drugs should also be ready. Epinephrine is not used because it enhances the effects of calcium infusion by increasing Ca^{++} current into the myocardial cell during the plateau phase of the action potential. When administered alone with Ca^{++}, it may produce potentially fatal arrhythmias.

Hypercalcemia

A hypercalcemic state exists whenever the total serum concentration of calcium rises to a value greater than 12 mg/dl. Increased ECF levels of Ca^{++} cause a greater diffusion gradient whereby the ion can move passively into cells. Of course, cells respond by increased active transport of Ca^{++} out of the cell, but this process can become quickly saturated and also requires considerable energy expenditure by the cell. Because of calcium's physiologic effects on the cell membrane, less Na^+ is able to diffuse into the cell through the competitive action of Na^+ and Ca^{++} on cell receptor sites. Furthermore, the internal membrane's effects on phospholipid and membrane proteins cause the membrane to become more rigid. Its entire permeability is changed. Enzymatic activities, secretory functions, and receptor integrity may all be disturbed in the presence of excess Ca^{++} in the ECF.

Such an altered membrane naturally behaves differently when it is excited. Depolarization is more difficult because less Na^+ can move into the cell. The cellular threshold for firing an action potential becomes more difficult to reach as threshold is made more positive whereas the resting membrane potential (RMP) is unaffected. Many of the symptoms of hypercalcemia therefore are due to cell membrane refractoriness to excitation.

Hypercalcemia is a symptom of underlying disease. The most common disorder that results in hypercalcemia is hyperparathyroidism, in which the gland produces excessive amounts of PTH. The hormone stimulates bone resorption, resulting in increased ECF concentration of Ca^{++} and decreased concentration of phosphate. Since the diseases may also be associated with poor regulation of excessive PTH output, there is little regulatory control over the hormone release in response to the serum concentration of Ca^{++}. Most cases of primary hyperparathyroidism are due to tumors of the parathyroid glands, which in the great majority of persons are benign adenomas. Surgical removal is usually indicated. This often results in the subsequent development of hypocalcemia, which is treated with oral calcium salts, vitamin D, and often magnesium. If healthy parathyroid tissue is present, it may be able to increase its output with time and eventually to assume complete control of the serum levels of Ca^{++}.

Other causes of hypercalcemia include malignant tumors of many different tissues, especially of the breast. Bone metastasis may often result in breakdown of normal bone and excessive Ca^{++} release, but hypercalcemia can occur in patients without metastasis to the skeletal system, and it seems probable that the mechanism for hypercalcemia in these cases is due to hormonal activity of the tumor. Many tumors produce inappropriate hormones, and PTH has been shown to be released from various types of malignant tissue. The effects of excessive PTH cause increased bone resorption and a rise in the serum concentration of calcium.

An additional cause of hypercalcemia is excessive ingestion of vitamin D. Usually the patient has a history of oral overdosage of vitamin D for many months. The effects on Ca^{++} metabolism continue long after the vitamin D is stopped.

Other conditions that may produce hypercalcemia include sarcoidosis, the milk-alkali syndrome (because of long-term ingestion of large amounts of milk and absorbable antacids), hyperthyroidism, Addison's disease, and various bone diseases.

Immobilization for long periods, particularly in children, may result in excessive bone resorption, hypercalcemia, and a state of osteoporosis, which is the result of a reduction in bone mass. It appears that stress and strain on bone as the result of normal muscular activity is a requirement for normal bone resorption-accretion balance. This may be due to the effects on the normal electrical field in bone, which in turn affects the activity of osteoclasts. It appears also that the skeletal system of an immobilized individual is less responsive to PTH. The effect of immobility is very rapid in its development; increased bone resorption occurs within a few days and continues as long as the immobility continues.

Signs and symptoms. Decreased neuromuscular irritability constitutes the basis for the signs and symptoms of hypercalcemia. Many systems of the body may be affected. The patient may have vague complaints, initially or in mild hypercalcemia. These complaints include fatigue, loss of interest in one's work, change in personality, and listlessness. In more severe cases the effects on the central nervous system are often more profound. The patient may develop headaches and excessive sleepiness and may eventually lapse into a comatose state. There is usually an associated skeletal muscle weakness of varying degrees, and occasionally paralysis may occur. The gastrointestinal tract often is affected, and decreased motility and secretion are the result. General abdominal pain and anorexia are often present, and occasionally nausea and vomiting are included. If the problem has been of long standing, there may also be a history of weight loss. Occasionally patients with hypervitaminosis D have diarrhea, but the mechanism for this development is unknown. Many times the patient with acute hypercalcemia is dehydrated, usually as the result of polyuria. This symptom is produced through the effects of a high Ca^{++} concentration on the renal tubular concentrating mechanism, particularly on the Na^+ transport mechanisms in the nephron. The mechanism for this effect is unknown. The hypercalcemic state will also cause excessive calcium excretion in the urine. As the solubility product for the $CaHPO_4$ reaction is exceeded, calcium salts are deposited throughout the tubules and collecting ducts of the kidney's nephrons. Nephrolithiasis (presence of kidney stones) is the eventual result, and probably all patients with recurrent kidney stones should be evaluated for hypercalcemia. Another system that is affected is the cardiovascular system. Symptoms may be produced in several different ways. Calcium salts may be deposited in the aorta and arterial walls, causing increased total peripheral resistance to blood flow. Furthermore, renal disease may complicate the clinical picture. Thus hypertension is seen in many patients with long-standing hypercalcemia. Calcification of other organs is certainly a possibility as well; for example, the eye is often affected by calcification (band keratopathy) of the cornea.

Changes in cardiac function also may occur. Calcium excess may increase the strength of contraction, and ECG changes, including depression of the T wave and a shortened Q-T interval, may also be recognizable.

Assessment and treatment

History. Attention to the patient's account of vague lethargy and personality changes is necessary when hypercalcemia is suspected. These symptoms often develop slowly and may be present for several weeks or months before the patient seeks help. Occasionally such individuals may actually be under psychiatric care for their problems, which eventually are shown to be entirely related to hypercalcemia. The review of systems is important, since hypercalcemia can produce pathologic changes in nearly every system of the body. Particular attention should be paid to the gastrointestinal tract, the renal system, and the neuromuscular system.

Neuromuscular assessment. The generalized muscle weakness of hypercalcemia is due to electrical changes in the cell membrane. Therefore all excitable cells may be affected. The deep tendon reflexes are usually hypoactive, and muscle tone and strength are diminished. Since another finding may be decreased hearing, the Rinne, Weber, and Schwabach tests should be performed. Careful examination of the eye is also necessary because both a diminished degree of visual acuity (related to problems in focusing caused by muscle weakness) and band keratopathy may be present. Determination of the intactness of the six cardinal positions of gaze, the ophthalmoscopic examination, and the use of Snellen's chart are therefore all indicated in the assessment of this patient. Band keratopathy appears as corneal opacities with denser centers. There may also be conjunctival densities and inflammatory changes in the conjunctiva. The patient may complain of itching or of the sensation of having a foreign body in the eye.

Gastrointestinal assessment. Auscultation of the abdomen in the hypercalcemic patient often will show diminished bowel sounds in all quadrants. Palpation may result in tenderness in all quadrants, and in some patients even light palpation will be exquisitely painful. The abdominal examination is important to rule out an acute abdominal condition.

Integumentary assessment. The skin is examined to determine whether dehydration is present. Skin turgor is assessed by pinching the skin over the sternum and noting the resiliency of this skin. In dehydration the skin remains folded and only slowly returns to normal. The skin should also be assessed for calcification, which will produce usually round, cystic lesions. They will cause sometimes severe itching, and secondary excoriations of the skin may be present.

Renal assessment. The renal assessment must include urinalysis to determine the specific gravity, which may be low, and the presence of protein, crystals, sediment, and glucose. The latter four findings may all be present in the patient with hypercalcemia. A 24-hour urine test for calcium clearance is also routinely performed. The renal assessment should also include determination of the presence of costovertebral angle (CVA) tenderness. This sign may be present, and the patient may also complain of deep bilateral flank pain during palpation. It is important to establish whether renal damage has occurred and whether any renal failure is present.

Skeletal system. Many patients with hypercalcemia will have bone disease known as *osteitis fibrosa cystica.* It is usually mild and is seen in the patient with primary hyperparathyroidism of long standing. Palpation of the bones is therefore done to determine whether any lesions or tenderness is present. However, the condition is not usually severe enough to produce measurable signs and symptoms and may show up only on x-ray films of the bones and teeth. Radiographic examination of the skeletal system is therefore usually necessary to establish the presence of this condition. The examiner should keep in mind that old or new fractures may be present if there have been significant bone resorption and osteoporotic changes.

Treatment. The treatment course of the patient with hypercalcemia is dependent on the degree of severity of the condition and the cause of the hypercalcemia. If the serum Ca^{++} value approaches 16 to 17 mg/dl, there is often danger of profound central nervous system depression that may be life threatening. In this crisis situation the high serum concentration of Ca^{++} must be quickly lowered. This may be accomplished by administration of phosphate, which will bind the Ca^{++}, according to the following reaction:

$$Ca^{++} + Phosphate \rightleftarrows Calcium\ phosphate$$

For milder cases of hypercalcemia (less than 12 mg/dl), symptomatic treatment is first carried out. The patient is rehydrated if dehydration is present, and the serum concentration of Ca^{++} may be lowered through the administration of normal saline solution in large amounts, along with a diuretic such as furosemide (Lasix), which inhibits tubular sodium reabsorption. The patient's fluid and electrolyte balance during this therapy obviously is of great importance. Hypervolemia is the most critical problem that can develop. The reason for the action of this regimen is that Na^+ and Ca^{++} movement occur together in the distal tubule, and ECF volume expansion results in excretion of Na^+ and Ca^{++}.

The underlying disorder, once identified, must be treated appropriately. Furthermore, it is worth noting that some conditions may be prevented through good patient education (such as milk-alkali syndrome and hypervitaminosis D) or excellent nursing care (such as immobilization effects).

CASE STUDY • PREGNANT WOMAN WITH TETANY

This case study represents a clinical situation in which hypocalcemia was due to a combination of several problems, rather than the result of a single disease state.

PAST HISTORY

A 38-year-old white woman presented in the emergency room of a local hospital with signs and symptoms of tetany. Pertinent history included previous surgery (appendectomy, dilatation and curettage, thyroidectomy, and adenoidectomy). Furthermore, 6 years previously the woman had had an intestinal bypass operation for exogenous obesity, after which she lost 140 pounds. The patient was pregnant for the ninth time and was nearly at term. The history suggests several possible causes for hypocalcemia. The surgical bypass of the duodenum would interfere with calcium absorption, which is dependent on fat-soluble vitamin D. In bypasses there is little fat absorption, since most takes place in the upper small intestine and is dependent on lipase, which is secreted into the duodenum from the pancreas. An additional problem at this point is of course the pregnancy.

PRESENT ILLNESS

This pregnancy was accompanied by several electrolyte problems, including hypomagnesemia, hypocalcemia, and hypokalemia. She was treated with K^+, Mg^+, and Ca^{++} supplementation during the pregnancy. The laboratory data (blood studies) at the time of admission showed the following:

$$Ca^{++} = 6.4 \text{ mEq/liter}$$
$$K^+ = 3.4 \text{ mEq/liter}$$
$$Na^+ = 142 \text{ mEq/liter}$$
$$Cl^- = 113 \text{ mEq/liter}$$
$$CO_2 = 19 \text{ mM/liter}$$
$$\text{Albumin} = 3.5 \text{ gm/dl}$$

The patient complained of tingling in her hands, face, and arms, which had started during the previous 8 hours. Just before coming to the emergency room her hands had gone into carpal spasm. She was unable to straighten her hands and cried out in pain when the physician attempted to straighten them. The vital signs were as follows:

Temperature: 36.1° C (97° F)
Pulse: 100 beats/min
Respirations: 28/min
Blood pressure: 120/88

The physical examination was within normal limits for a pregnant woman in the ninth month, except for 3+ deep tendon reflexes and a positive Chvostek's sign. Fetal heartbeat and movements were detectable.

TREATMENT

In the emergency room the patient received 2 ampules of calcium gluceptate in a solution of 5% dextrose in water. The serum concentration of calcium after this was 7.5 mEq/liter. The patient was admitted with an IV solution of 5% dextrose in water. The solution contained six ampules of calcium gluceptate in 1 liter of solution. Three hours after first having been seen in the emergency room, the patient developed generalized tetany, had a grand mal convulsion, and complained of pain with any movement. The IV solution was infusing at a rate of 125 ml/hr. About an hour later the patient was able to extend her right forefinger, although her hands were still in carpal spasm. During the next hour she was able to open her hand completely and within the following hour was out of bed and walking about. At this time the concentration of calcium in the IV solution was increased to 10 ampules/1000 ml, and within 3 hours the patient went into labor, delivering a normal baby girl. During the course of the 5-hour labor the serum concentration of calcium was measured and found to be 12.1 mEq/liter, and the potassium level went down to 2.3 mEq/liter. The infant's cord blood also indicated hypercalcemia and hypokalemia. The mother was treated with dextrose, 5%, in half-strength normal saline solution, with 40 mEq/liter of potassium chloride added. The serum electrolytes returned to normal during the next 24 hours, and the patient recovered and was discharged with her baby 4 days later. She was discharged on a regimen of potassium, calcium, and magnesium supplementation and triamterene (Dyrenium).

10

Other electrolyte imbalances

This chapter discusses the relatively rare electrolyte disorders that may only occasionally be encountered in the clinical situation. Often these electrolyte disorders are combined with more common problems of fluid, electrolyte, or acid-base balance, and therefore any specific symptomatology may be masked by other symptoms. The two major conditions to be described are chloride imbalance and magnesium imbalance. Trace metals of relevance and other electrolytes will be only briefly discussed.

CHLORIDE IMBALANCE

Chloride is the major anion of both the ICF and the ECF. Its major role is to balance cations in the cells and ECF. It does play a part in maintenance of the resting membrane potential (RMP), as previously discussed. Most cells are impermeable to chloride, but the anion can diffuse across most membranes in response to electrical and chemical gradients. The diffusion is, however, much slower than that of potassium. Chloride movement is necessary for normal carriage of CO_2, by participating electrically in the chloride shift (described on p. 105 and illustrated in Fig. 5-1). Transport across the cell membrane is passive, but there is evidence that a carrier mechanism may be involved, thus allowing for facilitated diffusion. This phenomenon has been shown to occur in erythrocytes, which are the cells participating in the chloride shift. The balance of chloride is maintained through renal excretion and reabsorption. The concentration of chloride in the urine ranges between 110 and 250 mEq/24 hr. The excretion of chloride is largely related to the dietary intake, which tends to be high in the typical American diet, since chloride accompanies sodium.

Chloride balance is related to bicarbonate ion (HCO_3^-) concentration, since the latter is the second most common body anion, being present in the ECF at a concentration of 24 mEq/liter. Preservation of electroneutrality requires an inverse relationship between HCO_3^- and chloride ion (Cl^-). When an abnormal increase in bicarbonate occurs, such as in compensation for respiratory acidosis, the Cl^- concentration decreases. The reverse situation also may occur when bicarbonate decreases, or conversely, Cl^- concentration may vary with HCO_3^- concentration.

The plasma concentration of chloride changes with relation to the water concentration in the ECF. Therefore dilutive hypochloremia may be seen in states of water excess, and water deficit will cause a concentrating effect on the plasma chloride.

The regulation of chloride concentration is determined by tubular reabsorption, since chloride is filtered at a concentration equal to that of plasma at the glomerulus. Reabsorption of chloride is dependent on cation (largely sodium) reabsorption. Since sodium reabsorption is under the control of aldosterone in the distal convoluted tubule (DCT) and collecting ducts, the chloride concentration in plasma and ECF is secondarily influenced by sodium reabsorption.

Hypochloremia

Loss of total body chloride can occur when gastric secretions, which are high in chloride, are lost from the body, as in prolonged vomiting or excessive nasogastric or fistula drainage. The newborn infant may develop hypochloremia as a sequela of diarrhea. One other common cause of this condition is diuretic therapy, which may deplete the body of various electrolytes including chloride.

When extracellular chloride concentration drops below 95 mEq/liter, the kidneys respond by reabsorbing proportionately more bicarbonate. The excess bicarbonate reacts with H^+ and drives the equation toward the formation of carbonic acid and CO_2 and water. This reaction will cause a drop in the ECF concentration of H^+, which results in metabolic alkalosis. In actuality, this condition may already be present, since most causes of hypochloremia are also associated with excessive H^+ loss. The excessive HCO_3^- reabsorption is accompanied by potassium and hydrogen secretion and loss in the urine; thus the metabolic alkalosis may be combined with production of an acid urine and a state of hypokalemia. The correction of metabolic alkalosis associated with hypochloremia is restoration of chloride stores through the administration of sodium chloride.

Hyperchloremia

Excess extracellular chloride is seen when ECF bicarbonate values drop, as in conditions in which the base bicarbonate decreases (metabolic acidosis). The fall in the buffer base, which is being utilized to buffer excessive H^+, causes increased chloride reabsorption. The classification and etiology of hyperchloremic and normochloremic metabolic acidosis are discussed in more detail in Chapter 5.

There is no single set of signs and symptoms for hypochloremia or hyperchloremia, since generally these electrolyte disturbances are associated with acid-base problems and are unlikely to exist as separate clinical entities.

MAGNESIUM IMBALANCE

Magnesium is an essential component of the human diet and is well conserved by the body. There are several important functions of magnesium, most of which are related to its activity as a common cofactor in enzymatic reactions. Several ATPase activities require ionized magnesium (Mg^{++}), and DNAases, hexokinase, and alkaline phosphatases may need this metal cation to function adequately. Magnesium also participates in neuromuscular excitability and is commonly used in preeclamptic patients to prevent convulsions. Magnesium appears to act at the synapse, decreasing transmission and depressing muscular irritability. It produces its sedative effect by blocking the release of the neurotransmitter acetylcholine. It appears also to have direct effects on the muscle cell excitability.

The many enzymatic reactions in which magnesium participates may proceed in the presence of manganese as well. These two ions are able to substitute for each other to a great degree. Calcium also interacts with the systems affected by magnesium, but it often opposes the action of magnesium and actually inhibits the enzymatic reaction. Calcium and magnesium also cross the cell membrane of many cells in a linked, or coupled, manner, with calcium extrusion being linked to magnesium entry. This active transport pump requires ATP and functions to maintain the comparatively higher intracellular magnesium concentration and to extrude excess calcium that has diffused into the cell.

Magnesium concentration is usually well maintained, and thus states of altered magnesium concentration are unusual and are often associated with serious pathophysiology. Magnesium deficiency or excess usually produces symptoms that reflect altered neuromuscular function.

Hypomagnesemia

A state of magnesium deficiency is present when the serum concentration drops below 1.5 mEq/liter, the normal value being between 1.5 and 2.5 mEq/liter. The condition can develop when intake is inadequate, absorption is impaired, or excretion is increased. Causes of hypomagnesemia are as follows:

1. Inadequate intake
   a. Malnutrition
   b. Alcoholism
2. Inadequate absorption
   a. Diarrhea, vomiting, nasogastric drainage, fistulas
   b. Excessive dietary calcium (competes with magnesium for transport sites)
   c. Diseases of the small intestine accompanied by malabsorption
   d. Hypoparathyroidism
3. Excessive loss
   a. Thiazide diuretics
   b. Aldosterone excess
   c. Polyuria

Signs and symptoms of hypomagnesemia are in some ways like those of hypocalcemia. Neuromuscular and cardiovascular functioning is the most disturbed, with patients suffering from muscle cramps and tetanic spasms, psychologic changes, hypotension and tachycardia, occasionally arrhythmias, abnormal sensations, ataxia, convulsions.

The treatment of the patient is by administration of magnesium salts intravenously or intramuscularly.

Hypermagnesemia

Hypermagnesemia is also an unusual clinical state, manifested by a serum concentration of magnesium greater than 2.5 mEq/liter. The most common cause of this condition is renal failure, although it can also be seen in patients receiving high doses of parenteral magnesium. An additional cause is hyperparathyroidism, since parathyroid hormone acts similarly on both calcium and magnesium.

Hypermagnesemia also affects cardiovascular and neuromuscular function. Since it can produce sympathetic ganglia blockade through inhibition of acetylcholine release from the preganglionic sympathetic neuron, vascular regulation becomes disturbed, and patients are subject to bradycardia and hypotension. The vasodilatory action of excess magnesium produces flushing, a sensation of warmth, and a variety of systemic problems in various areas of functioning, including nausea, vomiting, and drowsiness. Furthermore, the neuromuscular sedation may result in behavioral changes, lethargy, decreased reflexive activity, respiratory center depression and weakness of the respiratory muscles, and death by cardiac or respiratory arrest.

The treatment is directed at removing the excess magnesium by dialysis or by administering calcium, which counteracts magnesium in some physiologic functions.

IMBALANCE OF TRACE METALS AND TRACE ELEMENTS

The importance of trace metals and elements in normal human physiology cannot be denied, but characterization of deficiency or excess states is extremely difficult. In many cases the requirements are not known, and often there are various individual factors that complicate identification of both the requirements and the results of inadequate or excess amounts. Furthermore, there has been much recent research on little-known trace substances that appear to have significant effects on physiology and pathophysiology. Definitive statements with regard to some of these substances, such as selenium, vanadium, and molybdenum, cannot be made at the present time. Some of these substances exist as electrolytes at normal body pH, and others do not. Their overall role in fluid and electrolyte balance or imbalance is still the subject of research. Data regarding the major trace metals are provided in Table 10-1. Their requirements, normal concentrations, and physiologic functions, as well as effects of excesses of deficiencies, are tabulated.

The following trace elements are known to be required for metabolism and are generally involved in enzymatic function:
1. Molybdenum
2. Selenium
3. Vanadium
4. Cobalt
5. Chromium
6. Fluorine

Fluorine is not truly a required trace element but does prevent tooth decay when added to the diet in the form of fluoride. Several other, lesser-known trace metals are currently under investigation in many labora-

Table 10-1. Common trace metals and their functions

Trace metal	Function	Normal concentrations	Daily requirements	Physiologic effects	
				Excesses	Deficiencies
Iron	80% in molecules of hemoglobin; also a cofactor or component of several enzymes	35 mg/kg 50 mg/kg	5-10 mg/24 hr	Hemosiderosis in genetically susceptible individuals	Iron deficiency anemia
Copper	Requires for many enzymatic functions Used in melanin formation, bone development, myelin production, phospholipid synthesis, erythrocyte maturation	75-150 mg	2 mg/24 hr	Rare (can occur in Wilson's disease) Causes liver damage, lenticular degeneration, neurologic and renal pathology	Anemia Ataxia
Zinc	Cofactor or component of several enzymes (including carbonic anhydrase) Required for normal embryonic organogenesis Required for insulin release Involved in retinal function	2 gm	10-15 mg/24 hr	None known	Skin lesions Skeletal anomalies Decreased wound healing Dwarfism Hepatomegaly Hypogonadism
Manganese	Cofactor for several enzymes Required for normal bone growth, nervous irritability, lipid metabolism		6-8 mg/24 hr		
Iodine	Required in formation of thyroid hormones	25-50 mg	100-140 μg/24 hr	None known	Goiters Cretinism Thyrotoxicosis Thyroid tumors

tories, and identification of new requirements is probable within the next several years.

CASE STUDY • RENAL DIALYSIS PATIENT WITH ALTERED TASTE SENSATION

This case study describes the rare phenomenon of zinc deficiency. There are populations at risk for the development of such a deficiency even in the United States. Included are groups with very poor diets, in which the food contains less than 11 mg of zinc daily. Also at risk for the development of zinc deficiency are patients receiving total parenteral nutrition; patients with various disorders, including liver disease, malabsorption syndromes, and sickle cell disease; and some patients who have undergone intestinal bypass surgery. The deficiency has been recognized as causing hypogeuesthesia, or a decrease in taste, as one of the major manifestations. Decreased cellular immunity, anorexia, and poor growth are other problems that may develop. This case study describes a client on a regimen of renal dialysis who developed zinc deficiency.

IDENTIFYING DATA

Mr. L., a 35-year-old white man, was the victim of polycystic kidney disease. Both kidneys had been surgically removed 5 years before this episode. Mr. L. was maintained on a regimen of renal dialysis, which was done three times weekly in the community dialysis center.

PRESENT ILLNESS

Mr. L. has been slowly losing weight for about 6 months and complaining of anorexia. He stated that food tasted bitter or bland and was generally unappetizing. He would force himself to eat but occasionally was not able to eat at all. His wife had tried various ways of preparing his salt-free diet but was becoming increasingly frustrated, stating that the food tasted fine to her.

Mr. L. underwent tests of various types for possible malignant disease, but these were negative. He had complained of frequent upper respiratory infections and general fatigue as well. When no active disease was found, serum and hair zinc determinations were made. The values for zinc concentration are given below:

Hair: 125 ppm (normal, 180 ppm)
Serum: 60 mg/dl (normal, 75 mg/dl)

TREATMENT

Mr. L. began taking an oral zinc preparation ($ZnSo_4$ capsules, 220 mg daily). Within 3 weeks he began to increase his caloric intake as well as the amount of meat eaten daily. His taste sensation had returned to normal after a month, and he described eating as once again an enjoyable undertaking. His hair and serum zinc levels were normal, and he continued receiving zinc supplementation.

•   •   •

Implications of the case study are that many groups of nursing clients should be assessed for hypogeuethesia or dysgeuethesia. The elderly in particular may suffer from a borderline deficiency because of dietary and metabolic inadequacies. A simple assessment technique is the preparation of salty, sweet, sour, and bitter solutions of at least four different concentrations. The solutions are then dropped on the patient's tongue, alternating with drops of water, and the patient is asked to describe the taste sensation. A complete nutritional assessment and dietary history should also be part of the evaluation.

11

Developmental aspects of fluids, electrolytes, acids, and bases

DEVELOPMENTAL GROUPS

This chapter has been written because nurses care for clients of all age groups. Remarkable physiologic differences do exist at various developmental stages of life, and these differences have great bearing on the susceptibility of an individual to certain disorders, as well as on the ability to cope with alterations in normal homeostasis. The same care cannot be planned for an elderly dehydrated patient as for an infant with the same condition. The body water compartments and gain and loss routes, the ability to maintain the steady state, and the regulatory mechanisms are all different. Thus all developmental groups have been included in the discussion, and an attempt has been made to point out the ways in which these individuals differ from each other with regard to fluid, electrolyte, and acid-base balance. The discussion will begin with the fetal period. The lives of premature infants are now being saved through intensive care medicine and nursing at ages and weights that classify these newborn infants as fetuses in many senses of that word. Such immature organisms are poorly able to maintain fluid, electrolyte, and acid-base balance. Nurses caring for these infants require a thorough understanding of the particular physiology of the premature infant. Furthermore, an understanding of fetal physiology will be helpful to the nurse caring for normal newborns and older infants, since many aspects of their fluid, electrolyte, and acid-base regulatory systems are still developing. The chapter will focus mainly on renal physiology, anthropometric differ-

211

ences, and the developmental changes occurring in the various regulatory systems of the body.

Childhood is a period sometimes neglected in textbooks of fluid and electrolyte balance, and yet problems are very common in this age group. The physiology of the growing child as it relates to fluids and electrolytes will be described and common childhood problems and diseases that can interrupt the fluid and electrolyte balance will also be discussed.

Adolescence is comparable to the fetal-neonatal period in terms of the magnitude of physiologic changes that occur. The onset of puberty and, in females, the beginning of the menstrual cycle affect the body fluids and electrolytes. How hormones alter fluid and electrolyte balance will therefore be the focus of the discussion of adolescence.

The adult childbearing years are also included as a developmental stage, and the physiologic changes that occur in pregnancy and that are capable of interrupting normal fluid and electrolyte homeostasis will be described. In addition, pathophysiologic interruptions occurring in the normal pregnancy and affecting this homeostasis will be discussed.

Senescence begins at about the age of 30 years. The discussion of this stage of life will focus on the effects of aging at the cellular, tissue, and organ levels and on fluid and electrolyte balance. Many different alterations are possible in aged persons, and their fragile steady state makes an understanding of senescent physiology extremely important to the nurse.

THE FETUS
General aspects

The fetal period is divided into three trimesters, during which the various organ systems are developing at different rates. Most of organogenesis is completed by the third month of fetal life, and maturation and growth take place during the last two trimesters and often even during the early infancy period (birth to 3 months of age), sometimes known now as the "fourth trimester." The ability of the fetus to maintain fluid and electrolyte balance is dependent on maturity, as well as on the integrity of the fetoplacental unit. The major excretory organ of the fetus in utero is the placenta, and as its function decays during late pregnancy, the fetal kidneys, skin, and gastrointestinal tract increasingly mature. However, the birth of an infant weighing less than 1000 gm creates many problems in terms of life support. Of course, the crucial cardiovascular, neurologic, and respiratory maintenance takes priority, but in the infant who survives, increasing attention must be placed on fluid, electrolyte, and acid-base maintenance. The organs involved in this balance are immature and fragile, and the infant is usually not capable of coping with any threat to this balance without medical and nursing assistance.

Fetal kidney

The fetus does not require functional kidneys for normal development to proceed in utero. This is also true of the gastrointestinal tract and the skin. None of these organs play a role in fetal excretion, since the excretory function of the placenta apparently is the only way that waste products of fetal metabolism are removed. This is not to say that these organs are not capable of excretory function. Rapid development occurs throughout the last trimester, and at birth the skin, gastrointestinal tract, and kidneys will all be able to function as excretory organs. Their performance is not as efficient as in the older child; nevertheless, the full-term infant is entirely capable of excretory function through all three organs. If the infant is born before these organs have reached their full maturational potential, there may be problems involving both excretion and maintenance of fluid, electrolyte, and acid-base homeostasis.

The kidneys develop during organogenesis in an interesting manner. Three developmental stages occur in the formation of the mature kidneys, including growth and later regression of two very primitive kidneys: the pronephros and the mesonephros. The earliest kidney, the pronephros, appears after about 3 weeks in the human embryo. This kidney is not actually capable of urine formation, but its early appearance and later regression appear to be required before the second kidney, the mesonephros, can develop. One small duct of the pronephros is retained and becomes part of the mesonephros. This mesonephric duct eventually forms the vas deferens, epididymis, and ejaculatory duct of the male reproductive system, and in the female it is utilized to form some reproductive structures as well. While the pronephros regresses, the mesonephros forms, making its first appearance at about 4 weeks of human embryonic life. The mesonephros, although still evolutionarily primitive, is capable of urine formation. It precedes the development of the metanephros by about 2 weeks and regresses as the functionally mature metanephros forms. This permanent kidney is located retroperitoneally in the lumbar area. As the organ matures it then moves up into the flank position it occupies in the fully matured infant. The metanephros is formed from two different embryonic tissues: the ureteral bud and the metanephric blastema. The ureteral bud forms the collecting system, and the metanephric blastema gives rise to Bowman's capsule, most of the glomerulus, and the tubules of the individual nephrons. The tubules then make connections with collecting ducts, resulting in an anatomically complete microstructure by approximately 12 to 16 weeks of gestation. Urine formation occurs from that time onward. This fetal urine is hypotonic and contains no nitrogenous waste products. It is of small volume (3.5 ml/hr) at 28 weeks of gestation, but as the fetus grows, the urine volume increases to a value of nearly 40 ml/hr. This volume actually drops in the newborn infant to between 0 and 3 ml/hr and later rises at about 12 days to 10 ml/hr. Urine formation appears to be related to the volume and composition of amniotic fluid, but little is known about how urine formation is regulated and what its importance is. Infants born with renal defects or absence of the kidneys (renal agenesis) characteristically have very little amniotic fluid.

Fetal gastrointestinal tract and skin

At birth the fetal gastrointestinal tract is sterile, as well as both anatomically and functionally immature. During the fetal period the role of gastrointestinal secretion and motility is unknown. The fetus does swallow amniotic fluid, and it is believed that this fluid is absorbed into the fetal circulation. The secretions of the gastrointestinal tract form the meconium stool, which is normally not excreted during the fetal period except in cases of fetal distress. Thus the gastrointestinal tract does not function in fetal excretion. However, the ability of the gastrointestinal tract to absorb and secrete develops during fetal life; motility is also demonstrable, but slower emptying is characteristic because of the decreased muscular development. At birth the gastrointestinal tract beings to colonize with the normal flora, and digestive enzymes are produced as food is ingested. Motility and emptying are decreased at birth. Large amounts of water are lost in the stool during the newborn period, as will be discussed shortly.

The fragile skin of the fetus is not capable of water or waste excretion. As maturation continues during the last trimester, the sweat glands enlarge, and at birth both sensible and insensible water loss can occur through the skin. However, during the fetal period the skin plays no role in excretion or in fluid and electrolyte balance.

INFANCY
The premature infant

Within the category of prematurity by date we must also include the infant who is small for gestational age. Such an infant is characterized by a proportionately greater total body water (TBW) and ECF as compared to the full-term infant. Table 11-1 shows the relationship of the TBW and ECF with age. It is apparent that the low-birth-weight infant has a proportionately greater TBW and ECF and that the ECF compartment decreases dramatically during the first week of life. Another important consideration is the lesser amount of adipose tissue in such an infant. Fat is important not only as an energy store but also as insulation, and it has a function in normal thermoregulation as well. Greater heat loss through the skin of the low-birth-weight infant will result in an increase in insensible water loss (IWL). A marked difference in IWL is observed in premature infants as compared to the normal full-term infant, as well as to older children and adults. The data are summarized in Table 11-2. This compartment of water loss, it should be recalled, is essentially pure water without electrolytes. IWL is increased by heat, such as that provided to these infants by phototherapy and radiant-heat cradles, by metabolic increases (by as much as 20 ml/kg/24 hr), by variations in ambient temperature and humidity of the environment, by fever, and

Table 11-1. Developmental changes with age

Age group	TBW (%)	ECF (%)	ICF (%)
Low-birth-weight infant	90	65	35
Newborn	70-80	45	55
6 mo	65-70	35	65
16 yr to adult	60	25	75

Table 11-2. Insensible water losses

Age group	Amount (ml/kg)
Low-birth-weight infant	60-70
Newborn	60
6 mo	40
16 yr to adult	15-20

by increased respiratory rate. Furthermore, the physiologic and anatomic characteristics of the low-birth-weight infant dictate a proportionately greater IWL as compared to that of the normal newborn. Some of these characteristics include the greater ratio of surface area to volume in the smaller infant, the immaturity of the skin regulation over evaporative losses, and the greater vascularity of the skin.

Thus the premature infant is threatened by several types of fluid, electrolyte, and acid-base imbalance. A major one is dehydration caused by the contraction of the ECF in the first days of life, the increased IWL, the higher metabolism, and the heated environment. Almost invariably such an infant needs to be carefully watched for signs of dehydration (Chapter 6), and parenteral fluids are often required. Many very small infants are not able to suck adequately, and the small gastric volumes they are able to tolerate through gavage feedings are not adequate to maintain or repair fluid, electrolyte, and glucose deficits. The amount required is dependent on the urine volume and the specific gravity of the urine. The latter is a measure of the concentrating ability of the kidneys, which is often decreased greatly in the low-birth-weight infant. The urine output should be maintained between 1 and 3 ml/kg/hr. The IWL must be taken into account in estimating the amount of fluids the infant requires. The weight must also be very closely monitored, since it may be the only sign of impending dehydration or even of more serious problems such as metabolic acidosis (see the case study at the end of Chapter 5). The usual amount of parenteral fluid needed by the low-birth-weight infant maintained in an incubator is 75 to 100 ml/kg/24 hr, the fluid usually containing potassium, calcium, and 10% to 12% glucose. This fluid provides the calories required for tissue anabolism in the infant, providing that the infant is able to metabolize glucose at the usual rate of between 5 and 10 mg/kg/24 hr.

A complication of administering glucose-containing IV fluids to low-birth-weight infants is hyperglycemia. The reason lies in several factors, such as an inability of the infant to metabolize the infused glucose, a lower tubular maximum (T_m) in the renal tubules, and a decreased release of insulin or possibly tissue insensitivity to insulin. The resultant glycosuria provokes an osmotic diuresis, causing further water loss and dehydration in infants already at risk.

Another common problem experienced by the low-birth-weight infant is acidosis, resulting from hypoxia experienced during labor, delivery, or the postnatal period. The cause of the acidosis is both respiratory insufficiency and increased metabolic demands for oxygen, which eventually result in anaerobic metabolism and acidosis. Many factors contribute to the acidosis, which must be viewed in part as physiologic, the normal arterial pH of the neonate being 7.30. One of these factors is renal immaturity, which results in less acidification of the urine and less bicarbonate reabsorption. The fetal circulation is abolished, and vascular shifts and lung expansion, along with increases in the pulmonary vascular diameters and drops in resistance, also occur during this crucial period of life. There is also a variable metabolic rate of the newborn, depending on whether the child is handled or perhaps circumcised in the delivery room, cold stressed, or subjected to other environmental stresses.

The full-term neonate is usually able to manage the acidosis, and normal pH and Pco_2 values are reached within 24 hours. However, the low-birth-weight infant is more at risk for severe hypoxia and acidosis. The presence of stress, such as cold or heat stress, and the high incidence of respiratory distress syndrome in the premature infant also predispose him to acidosis. Furthermore, this infant is subject to delayed metabolic acidosis caused by renal hypoxia at birth. The latter leads to renal failure with subsequent acidosis, hypervolemia, and acidosis, which may occur several days or weeks after the birth.

The normal newborn

There are special aspects of neonatal physiology that make the fluid, electrolyte, and acid-base balance unique and delicate. The anatomic characteristics, as well as the physiologic immaturity, of the newborn and older infant dictate much higher risks for imbalance than are seen in older children or adults.

Anatomic and physiologic considerations

The greatest anatomic difference in infants relates to the relationship of surface area to volume. Because of the relatively greater size of the head and other factors, the ratio of surface area to volume is greater, and this implies that the infant has more surface from which to lose water and to lose or gain heat. Therefore the IWL is proportionately greater, as was shown in Table 11-2. On a percentage basis, the infant's TBW is greater than that of older children and adults. The smaller the infant, the greater the percentage of TBW to weight. In the normal newborn about 80% of the weight is due to the water content. In the adult this value is closer to 60% but is dependent on the amount of adipose tissue present, which will cause the percentage of TBW to be lower. Another important variable in fluid loss and gain is the basal metabolic rate

(BMR), which is three times higher in infancy than in adulthood. The high BMR is a result of the growth that is characteristic of this developmental stage and the great metabolic demands of a proportionately larger and growing brain; thus the infant requires a greater number of kilocalories per kilogram. The newborn requirement is about 110 kcal/kg, compared to the adult needs of 48 kcal/kg, depending of course on illness, exercise, and stress. The child's needs are also somewhat variable because the presence of fewer or acute illness generally increases the BMR and the energy requirements. That the BMR is nearly three times the adult value has important implications for fluid and electrolyte balance. The water of oxidation, which is produced through the electron transport system of the mitochondria, is greater in amount in the child, since 10 ml/100 kcal is produced this way. Furthermore, it is through metabolism of foodstuffs that metabolic wastes that must be excreted daily are produced. This solute load must be excreted through the kidney with an adequate urinary output. The concentrating ability of the neonatal kidney is less than that of the older child's kidney, and therefore a proportionately greater amount of water must be excreted with this solute load. Thus the water loss through the kidneys is also greater than in the adult, in terms of milliliters per kilograms. These data are summarized in Table 11-3. Another problem that may arise in infancy is caused by the decreased glomerular filtration rate (GFR). Recall that this value is about 120 ml/min in adults. It is difficult to measure in infants but is less than 30 ml/min. This low rate is probably due to a combination of several factors, such as the lowered arterial blood pressure in the newborn and the functional immaturity of the filtering membrane. Infants are also refractory to the effects of antidiuretic hormone (ADH), and this may play a role in the decreased concentrating ability of the nephron. Infants do not seem as well able to handle sodium imbalances, and they tend to retain proportionately more sodium if it is present in either the formula or the breast milk. Sodium retention results in expansion of the ECF, and it is possible that the greater percentage of ECF in infants (45%) compared to adults (18%) is due to inadequate sodium excretion.

Turnover of the body fluids is also very different in infants. The entire ECF is replaced every 3 days in small infants, in the sense that the infant loses nearly 600 ml/24 hr from water-loss compartments. Compared to the infant's total ECF of 1500 ml, this fluid loss is over one third of the ECF. In an adult about 2400 ml of fluid is lost from the body each day. This amount represents only one sixth of the ECF.

Overall fluid loss in the infant, as illustrated in Table 11-4, shows

Table 11-3. Urine output changes (by age)

Age	Urine output (ml/hr)
Low-birth-weight infant	Less than 1
Newborn	1
12-day-old infant	10
6 mo	12
16 yr	35

Table 11-4. Water-loss route changes (by age)

Water-loss compartment	6 mo (ml/kg)	16 yr (ml/kg)
IWL	40	20
Urinary system	50	25
Gastrointestinal system	5	2.5
TOTAL	95	47.5

proportionately greater water loss per kilogram of body weight, but the tonicity of these fluid losses is not greatly different from that of the adult. The effect is one of an overall greater fluid and electrolyte loss and therefore of greater proportionate water and caloric requirements. It also suggests that the steady state of the small infant is much more fragile than in the adult; that is, the regulatory and compensatory responses cannot operate as efficiently in the functionally immature organism.

A further consideration with regard to fluid and electrolyte balance is the dependence of children on adults for the meeting of their needs. The neonate or infant cannot express his need for fluids and is therefore more likely to become dehydrated or overhydrated if caretaking is inadequate.

The acid-base balance during infancy also differs significantly because of several factors. The ability of the infant to acidify the urine is decreased. However, it is important to keep in mind that the nitrogen balance of the growing organism differs from that of the adult, since protein anabolism far exceeds catabolism during growth. Therefore the nitrogenous waste load on the kidneys is far less, and the normal infant is well able to handle waste excretion. However, in states of metabolic or respiratory acidosis or alkalosis, compensation may not be as effective as in the adult. This is partly due to the lower renal threshold for HCO_3^-

reabsorption and to the inability to acidify the urine beyond the infant's steady state values. It should be recalled that the newborn is in a state of acidosis, with a blood pH of around 7.3. This acidosis is usually corrected during the first 24 hours of life. It is caused by the limited buffering capacity of the ECF, and several studies have shown that the major problem arises from the low HCO_3^- reabsorption characteristic of the newborn period. Therefore the neonatal acidosis is associated with a decreased HCO_3^- concentration in the plasma.

CHILDHOOD

The major phenomenon characterizing childhood is growth of long bones, tissues, and organs in a sequential, irreversible pattern that is highly predictable. Of course, the childhood period is also characterized by development of immunocompetence, and thus the child suffers frequent infectious disease. Both the growth phenomenon and the common illnesses of childhood are associated with specific fluid, electrolyte, and acid-base problems.

Growth

Growth proceeds, along with further differentiation and maturation of the various organ systems involved in maintenance of the steady state. The kidneys grow in size and volume, and there is an increase in the number of glomeruli, with results in an increase in filtering surface from 0.2 m^2 at birth to 1.6 m^2 in adolescence. The renal system, for example, develops the ability to increase the GFR over several years, so that adult values are reached by late childhood or early adolescence. Renal blood flow (RBF), ability to respond to a salt load, acidification properties, bicarbonate reabsorption, and ability to concentrate the urine are all properties that develop during the childhood period, some more rapidly than others. With regard to the capacity of the child to respond to threats to fluid, electrolyte, or acid-base balance, the maxim is that the older the child, the better he is able to cope.

Bone growth, of course, contributes to the electrolyte balance of the growing organism, since large amounts of calcium and phosphate are required and are mobilized from the ECF into the crystallizing bone. Acid is released from bone during growth as the hydroxyapatite crystal is formed from calcium, phosphates, and water. Therefore the process of growth contributes acid to the ECF, and of course this acid must be buffered and excreted. For normal bone growth to proceed, an exogenous supply of calcium and phosphate is also necessary, as well as vitamin D formation in the skin. The requirements for these minerals are consequently higher during childhood.

Common fluid, electrolyte, and acid-base problems of childhood

A general rule with regard to childhood illnesses is that the regulatory and compensatory responses to imbalance are less stable and tend to operate within a more narrow range of alteration, with less tolerance for large changes in balance. The most common physical problems afflicting children are accidents, upper respiratory infections, gastrointestinal disturbances, congenital anomalies, and common infectious, exanthem-producing illnesses. Children frequently respond to illness with a fever of both higher temperature and greater duration than adults. Fever is a pathophysiologic process that can profoundly affect fluid, electrolyte, or acid-base balance and therefore deserves special consideration in this section.

Fever. Fever is defined as a significant elevation occurring in the core body temperature and caused by the effects of pyrogens. For an understanding of its significance it is necessary to review the thermoregulatory processes that maintain core temperature in both children and adults. Table 11-5 shows the normal regulation of core body temperature through centers in the hypothalamus. The existence of centers of heat loss and heat gain is postulated, with reciprocal innervation between them. When heat gain mechanisms are stimulated, there is inhibition of the heat loss center, and vice versa. The set point for normal core temperatures (37° C) is genetically determined and differs slightly among all individuals. It is also affected by circadian rhythmicity, being lower in the morning and higher in the evening. Temperature is further influenced by metabolism, and the high rate in children causes their basal body temperature to be somewhat greater than in adults. The hypothalamus is able to sense the body temperature and, in accordance with the set point, continually adjust heat loss and heat gain so as to maintain the value at the set point. These centers are known as the body "thermostat" and consist of set point–sensitive neurons, the so-called *thermoreceptors*, and the neurons of the heat loss and gain centers themselves. The thermoreceptors are able to directly measure the temperature of the blood and to feed this information into the heat loss and gain centers. There is also a widespread temperature-detecting system that supplies input into the hypothalamus. Pyrogens are believed to act by disturbing the thermoreceptors and by

Table 11-5. Heat loss and gain mechanisms

Heat loss mechanisms	Heat gain mechanisms
Vasodilation of skin vessels	Vasoconstriction of skin vessels
Sweating or panting; piloerection	Shivering; increased exercise
Decreased metabolism	Increased metabolism
Behavioral responses	Behavioral responses

"resetting" the set point to a higher than normal value. The result is that the heat loss centers are inhibited and the heat gain centers stimulated. The heat loss and heat gain mechanisms are summarized in Table 11-5.

The aim of heat loss mechanisms is to transfer the internal core heat to the periphery—that is, the skin—to dissipate this heat load from the body. Sweating, through evaporative heat transfer, is an efficient mechanism for this purpose, since 0.6 kcal(heat)/gm water is lost through the evaporation of sweat from the skin surface. Evaporation differs from radiation and convection, which require that the ambient temperature be less than the body temperature before heat transfer can occur. Sweating does not require a temperature gradient but is enhanced by a hot environment, particularly if the vapor pressure gradient from the skin to the air is great. The innervation of the sweat glands is through the sympathetic nervous system, which stimulates their activity. Heat loss is also aided by radiation and convection of heat from the skin. These mechanisms are enhanced by vasodilation of skin vessels and opening up of arteriovenous anastomoses, which normally act to shunt blood away from skin capillaries. The great surface area of the skin can thus be warmed, and if a heat gradient from skin to air is present, the heat will dissipate physically into the environment. Panting is also effective but is not an important response in man. There is also piloerection, which is contraction of the small muscles that regulate the hair follicles, causing the hair to "stand on end" and thus increasing the surface area over which heat loss can occur. Piloerection is not significant in humans. Behavioral responses in humans that aid in heat loss include the seeking of a cool environment and a decrease in the clothing worn.

Heat gain involves a shunting of blood to the internal core organs and a decrease in function of all heat loss mechanisms. For example, vasoconstriction, which causes less blood to move to the periphery, accounts for the chilled feeling of a person who has a fever. Shivering also effectively increases heat production, as does exercise. Increased metabolism will result in greater heat production, as exemplified by the higher body temperature of persons with hyperthyroidism and by the lower values in persons with hypothyroidism. The behavioral responses associated with heat gain are the seeking of a warm environment, the wearing of warmer clothes, and, in fever or in cold environments, the assumption of a curled-up fetal position, which decreases the surface area exposed to the environment and thus minimizes heat loss. Body temperature can be increased through infectious or inflammatory processes or through hyperthermic states (which will be discussed later). The febrile state associated with infections and inflammations is due to the release of endogenous pyrogen (EP) from involved cells. It is important to stress that a pyrogen is a product of the host's own cells, not a bacterial product. Thus endotoxins probably act mainly by stimulating the production of EP, which is apparently not a breakdown product of dead or dying cells but rather is actively produced by neutrophils and reticuloendothelial cells through metabolic pathways. Many authorities believe that EP acts on prostaglandin synthesis in the vessel walls of hypothalamic blood vessels, and the prostaglandin then directly acts to reset the hypothalamus. There is evidence, however, that prostaglandins are not always mediators of fever.

The effects of fever on fluid balance are related to the increased metabolism stimulated by the fever, which causes an increase in IWL of 10% for every degree Celsius of fever. There is often a great potential for drying out of the body tissues in fever, and dehydration is common. Furthermore, the usual treatment for EP-produced fever is antipyretic drugs, which reset the hypothalamic core temperature set point back to the normal value. The major mechanism for heat loss under these conditions is sweating; thus both fluids and electrolytes are lost. In small children with fever, the potential for dehydration is great, particularly if the fever is prolonged. One important developmental aspect of the febrile response to EP is related to the often-noted absence of fever in the newborn, even in the presence of major infections. It has been speculated that the absence of fever is due either to immaturity of the temperature regulation of neonates or to the possibility of refractoriness of the hypothalamus to EP, suggesting that fever is, immunologically speaking, a developmental response not present in early life. Neonates have a limited capacity for heat storage and rely in part on nonshivering thermogenesis for heat production, particularly when they are cold stressed. This mechanism takes place in the brown fat of newborns, which consists of collections of tissue between the scapulae, on the back of the neck, in the axillae, in the mediastinum, and around the kidneys. Heat production is high in brown fat because of the uncoupling of oxidative phosphorylation; thus the constraints of adenosine diphosphate (ADP) concentration on the rate of electron transport, and consequently on heat production, are removed. Thus nonshivering thermogenesis results in an increased oxygen consumption when the small infant is stressed by a cold environment.

Another developmental variable in thermoregulation is that the set point for body temperature appears to be lower in the premature or small-for-gestational-age infant. For this reason, such infants appear to be physiologically hypothermic, with normal set points below 36.5° C.

Contrasted with fever are states of hyperthermia, in which the body temperature is elevated because of disturbed heat loss rather than because of EP. The fluid and electrolyte problems in hyperthermic conditions are different from those in EP-produced fever. Such conditions as heat stroke, in which the core temperature elevates to values greater than 40.6° C (105° F), are usually seen in unacclimatized individuals exercising in a hot, humid environment. Several factors contribute to this hyperpyrexia, including the decreased vapor pressure gradient between the skin and the air, and the production of a large heat load through muscle exercise. Since this condition is often associated with cardiovascular signs of volume depletion, water and electrolyte loss must occur, but the ability of the sweating mechanism is nevertheless not efficient. The major deficiency appears to be water depletion with resultant hypernatremia. Hypokalemia is also often found.

Table 11-6 shows the pathophysiologic basis for the treatment of fever, indicating that "fever" as a symptom may arise from many causes and that treatment must be based on the particular thermoregulatory process that has been disrupted. Thus it is inappropriate to treat a patient with an antipyretic drug when the pathophysiology does not involve resetting of the hypothalamic set point. This is true for patients with malignant hyperthermia, heatstroke, hypernatremia (Chapter 7), burns, and conditions resulting from the use of certain drugs (aspirin, anticholinergics). The usual treatment is aimed at removing the excess heat from the body. This has important implications for the nursing care of patients with EP-produced fever. Traditional approaches, such as sponging with ice water or alcohol, giving ice water enemas, and using ice blankets, are aimed at removing heat. None of these measures are directed at the pathophysiology involved in the fever production, and in fact they will cause intense vasoconstriction as a direct effect of the cold. The cold stress will increase the BMR, which will result in even greater heat production and consequent discomfort. Shivering is a common response to sponging with cold water and will cause heat production. Further dangers are related to alcohol toxicity, especially in small infants and children, from inhalation during alcohol sponging. Ice water enemas may result in hyponatremia or hypothermia. The only acceptable use of such measures is in cases of extremely high temperature elevation in which convulsions or brain damage is imminent and antipyretic drugs have not yet taken effect. Tepid sponging is otherwise suggested if the child is not responding appropriately to the drugs administered. In this case the temperature gradient for heat loss still exists, without a threat of vasoconstriction. The child should be observed for any sign of cold stress and, at the first sign of shivering, removed to a warmer environment. It should be further emphasized that fever is rarely a dangerous threat to health except in infants under 1 year of age, in whom febrile convulsions are fairly common. Most fevers will break without treatment and without sequelae or threat to the patient's health.

Other nursing measures in the care of the febrile patient include observation of the hydration state and appropriate intervention to balance intake and output. Furthermore, the occasional problems of hypokalemia and hypernatremia should be assessed.

Fever is a reponse to illness and is characteristic of even mild illnesses in children. In fact, the ability of children to tolerate fever often amazes adults. Common childhood illnesses, as we have mentioned, include upper respiratory infections, which are often characterized by fever. Upper respiratory illness itself may disrupt fluid, electrolyte, and acid-base balance, independently of its fever-producing effects.

Upper respiratory infections. The range of upper respiratory infections is from mild colds through bacterial pneumonia, but some general principles hold true. Children with upper respiratory infections suffer some degree of impairment in oxygenation. Infants with extremely mild nasopharyngitis can become disproportionately dyspneic because of their inability to mouth breathe or because of the immaturity of the respiratory center's regulatory ability in handling mild hypoxia. This immaturity in some infants is speculated to contribute to the cause of sudden infant death syndrome. A major reponse in all children to respiratory embarrassment is increased rate and depth of breathing, resulting in an increased IWL through lung evaporation and possibly contributing to dehydration. An additional problem arises when diffusion of gases across the alveolar membrane is impeded—for example, because of accumulated inflammatory secretions. The child may become acutely

Table 11-6. Pathophysiologic basis for symptomatic treatment of fever*

Disease process causing fever	Pathophysiology of fever	Clinical findings	Appropriate non-specific treatment	Inappropriate non-specific treatment
Infection, malignancy, allergy, steroid fever, collagen disease	Endogenous pyrogen causes rise in hypothalamic set point	Patient complains of feeling cold; piloerection; cold extremities; absent or minimal sweating; body positioned to minimize surface area, shivering	Drug-induced lowering of hypothalamic set point (e.g., with aspirin, acetaminophen); supply sufficient clothing and covers for maximal comfort; avoid shivering	Physical removal of heat (e.g., sponging, ice blanket, ice water enemas); without change in set point these measures will cause discomfort, increase metabolic rate, and will only lower body temperature for brief period
CNS lesion, DDT poisoning, scorpion venom, radiation, epinephrine and norepinephrine overdose	Agent or illness acts directly on hypothalamus to raise set point	Same as above	Drug-induced lowering of hypothalamic set point theoretically indicated as above; it is not clearly established, however, as possible with presently available drugs	Same as above

Malignant hyperthermia, hyperthyroidism, hypernatremia, primary defect in energy metabolism, aspirin overdose	Heat production exceeds heat loss mechanisms	Patient complains of feeling hot; no piloerection; hot extremities; active sweating; body positioned to maximize surface area	Undress patient; physical removal of heat (e.g., ice blanket, sponging)	Attempt to lower set point (which is already set normally) with drugs (e.g., aspirin—possible toxicity of drug without potential benefit)
Overuse of sauna, exposure to industrial heat, overdressing	Environmental heat load exceeds normal heat loss mechanisms	Same as above	Eliminate heat source; undress patient; physical removal of heat is effective but is not usually necessary	Same as above
Ectodermal dysplasia, burns, phenothiazine anticholinergic overdose, heatstroke	Defective heat loss mechanisms cannot cope with normal heat load	Patient complains of feeling hot; sweating decreased (secondary to disease process); hot extremities; body positioned to maximize surface area	Provide cool environment; undress patient; physical removal of heat may be necessary	Same as above

*From Stern, R. C.: Pediatrics **59**:92, Jan., 1977. Copyright American Academy of Pediatrics.

hypoxic, and the PO_2 of the blood may fall while the PCO_2 rises. Respiratory compensation will occur but may be inadequate, resulting in respiratory acidosis. Furthermore, as the cells convert to anaerobic metabolism, metabolic acidosis will also be present. Thus the major problems in children with upper respiratory infections, with relation to fluids and electrolytes, are dehydration and acidosis.

Gastroenteritis. The third problem to be discussed is gastroenteritis. This condition develops commonly in children because of their immature immune system and their propensity for infections transmitted through the fecal-oral route. The major problem inherent in acute gastroenteritis, namely dehydration, was discussed in detail in Chapter 6. For many reasons, previously outlined, children are extremely susceptible to the development of dehydration when suffering from acute gastroenteritis. Another important consideration is that in infants the diarrhea may become intractable and chronic, and therefore these children are constantly at risk for both fluid and electrolyte problems and must be carefully assessed and treated. Recovery is possible now, with the use of hyperalimentation in the severe cases, so that the gastrointestinal mucosa can recover from the inflammatory damage and once again become sufficient.

The cause of gastroenteritis in children is believed to be usually viral, with less than 10% of cases resulting from actual bacterial food poisoning or infections. Thus the treatment is directed at the fluid, electrolyte, and acid-base imbalance. Initially the child is restricted to clear fluids or, if hospitalized, often receives nothing by mouth, with fluid replacement and repair being done parenterally. Many children require a rest period during which their gastrointestinal tracts can recover. Fluids may actually irritate and stimulate the gut, further enhancing the inflammation present. When fluids are administered intravenously, the repair fluids are estimated by the percentage of dehydration that is present. Therefore, for 5% dehydration, 50 ml/kg is necessary, for 10% dehydration, 100 ml/kg, and so forth. This fluid is usually an isotonic fluid to replace that lost through diarrhea or vomiting. If the IWL has been extensive, then hypotonic fluid is used to repair the volume deficit. For calculation of the amounts of water and electrolyte replacement that should be provided for the child with gastroenteritis, the following analysis, based on a body weight of 10 kg, is given.

Repair fluids for 10% dehydration. For a child weighing 10 kg, with a 10% loss of isotonic body fluids, 100 ml/kg is required. The fluid is usually administered more rapidly if the child shows signs of shock, or administration is spread over 2 days if not. Three fourths is administered during the first 24 hours; thus the child will require 750 ml for repair of the dehydration during the first day. The solution chosen should be isotonic.

Maintenance. The water and electrolyte compartments are basically the same as in the adult, but the proportionate amounts of loss are greater in children.

For IWL, the daily maintenance amount is 40 ml/kg and of course is adjusted upward if fever is present (10% for every degree Celsius). Therefore the child weighing 10 kg requires 400 ml/24 hr of water to replace that lost through IWL.

Since urinary losses are about 50 ml/kg, the water replacement needs amount to 500 ml/24 hr for the child weighing 10 kg.

Gastrointestinal losses, generally very small (5 ml/kg), increase to about 25 to 35 ml/kg in moderate diarrheal disease, and they are replaced with isotonic fluid because stool is very similar to ECF. The child requires 350 ml/24 hr as long as the diarrhea continues.

Summarizing the requirements. Daily replacement and repair needs of a child weighing 10 kg and with acute gastroenteritis are as follows:

Repair: 750 ml isotonic solution
IWL: 400 ml water
Urine: 500 ml water*
Gastrointestinal: 350 ml isotonic solution
TOTALS: 1100 ml isotonic solution
+ 900 ml water with 5% dextrose
2000 ml total fluid needs

The composition of this fluid is determined by estimating the fraction of the total that is isotonic and multiplying it by the usual amount of sodium in an isotonic solution (150 mEq/liter):

$$\frac{1100}{2000} \times 150 = 82.5 \text{ mEq Na}^+/\text{liter}$$

The major cation should be sodium until renal function is assured and the potassium (at around 30 mEq) can be added. An appropriate IV fluid for the first 24 hours is 0.45 NaCl in 5% dextrose in water. Often bicarbonate replaces some of the chloride anion because gastrointestinal secretions are high in bicarbonate. A solution such as half-strength Ringer's lactate solution is then appropriate.

---

*Urine is of course not pure water and does contain excess cations and anions, but for purposes of replacement these milliequivalents are disregarded.

ADOLESCENCE

The developmental stage of adolescence is marked by rapid, major changes in both anatomy and physiology. Growth rate increases greatly, and there is of course an increased metabolic demand at this time. A critical weight is reached in the young female (between 47.7 and 49.5 kg [106 to 110 lb]), at which time the menstrual cycle begins to become established. Males do not have a corresponding physiologic cycle of sexual function, but androgenic hormones are secreted in greater amounts, causing maturation of the secondary sex characteristics. In the female, however, unique cyclic physiologic changes occur with a periodicity of about 28 days. During this time many systems of the body are affected, and fluid and electrolyte balance changes in most women to some degree. Certain individuals have very disturbed function concomitant with the menstrual cycle. Therefore the normal menstrual cycle will be described, and then the fluid and electrolyte imbalances that may occur will be discussed.

Normal menstrual cycle

Fig. 11-1 diagrams the hormonal, ovarian, and endometrial changes that occur during the normal menstrual cycle. Notice that at the start of the cycle the hormones estrogen and progesterone begin to rise; estrogen peaks before progesterone, and then both reach a plateau, after which they drop sharply in serum concentration just before the menses. The plateau occurs in the luteal phase, during which the "premenstruum" is said to exist. In most susceptible females, it is at the premenstruum that fluid and electrolyte imbalances most commonly occur. The fall in estrogen and progesterone levels signals endometrial sloughing and bleeding, since these hormones support the endometrial growth in preparation for possible pregnancy. Once that hormonal support is withdrawn, the endometrium cannot be sustained, and menstruation begins.

During the premenstruum about 40% of all menstruating females experience the "premenstrual syndrome," which is characterized by a variety of signs and symptoms that may or may not all exist together. These include emotional lability, headaches, mastalgia, nausea, excessive thirst and appetite, sugar craving, edema, and weight gain. Some physiologic parameters that have been studied during the premenstruum include water and electrolyte balance, cognitive performance, and autonomic nervous system activity. With reference to the latter, it is well known that the phenomenon of autonomic system hypersensitivity occurs during the premenstruum. Other studies have shown alterations in special senses,

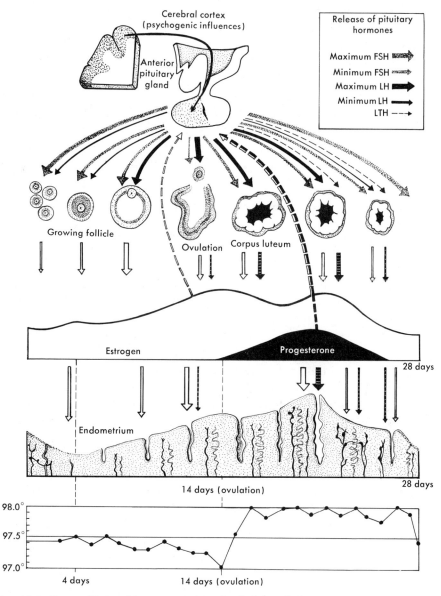

Fig. 11-1. Interrelationships among cerebral, hypothalamic, pituitary, ovarian, and uterine functions throughout a usual 28-day menstrual cycle. Variations in basal body temperature are also illustrated.

such as vision and hearing. Cognitive function does not appear to be significantly affected. Water and electrolyte changes in the normal menstrual cycle have not been extensively studied. There is some evidence that fluctuations in TBW do occur during the menstrual cycle. Weight gains generally appear to be small and often are not significant in the normal female, but there are individuals who suffer major changes in body water, which are evidenced as vascular headaches, perhaps related to cerebral edema, and swelling and bloating of the hands, feet, face, and abdomen. Most of these women also experience swings in emotion and often become seriously depressed. Accidents, illnesses, crimes committed by women, and suicides all occur more frequently during the premenstrual period.

Etiology of premenstrual fluid and electrolyte changes

The fluid and electrolyte changes that occur during the menstrual cycle are not well characterized, but retention of water does appear to occur in most women with the premenstrual syndrome. The cause of the water retention and resultant edema may be multifactorial. That the ratio of estrogen to progesterone changes during the menstrual cycle may be etiologic. There is some evidence that progesterone levels are low in women subject to the premenstrual syndrome, and progesterone has been used to treat the symptoms successfully. Estrogen is in part responsible for endometrial and breast hyperplasia and is known to increase the water content of the skin, but neither estrogen nor progesterone changes alone are sufficient to account for the premenstrual syndrome. Cyclic changes in both serum aldosterone and plasma renin activity have been shown to occur during the normal menstrual cycle, with peaks of concentration occurring during the luteal phase. In women with premenstrual syndrome these concentrations appear to be higher than normal. It is conceivable that aldosterone increases sodium and water retention, thus promoting increased TBW and edema. However, progesterone is also high at this time, and it is known to be natriuretic. The role of prostaglandins in premenstrual changes is now being characterized, and these substances are clearly implicated in dysmenorrhea. Perhaps they may also be involved in premenstrual fluid and electrolyte changes. Another substance of possible importance is prolactin. The premenstrual syndrome appears to occur with higher-than-normal frequency in women with vitamin B_6 deficiency, and vitamin B_6 appears to suppress prolactin, as does the drug bromocriptine. Patients with premenstrual syndrome are reported to respond well both to large doses of vitamin B_6 and also to bromocriptine.

Presumably both the vitamin-deficient patient and normal women suffering from premenstrual syndrome have excessive prolactin activity.

This interesting area of physiologic functioning is of great relevance to nursing care, since the responses of our patients to drugs and treatments, as well as their general susceptibility to disease, may be cycle dependent. Furthermore, since most nurses are female, changes related to the menstrual cycle may be a variable in the efficacy of our own role and functions.

YOUNG ADULTHOOD

Although many physiologic changes occur during the adult stage of life, most of them are related to the senescent process, which unfortunately begins to take place very early, perhaps even before the age of 30 years. However, a major developmental task associated with physiologic changes in the female is childbearing. Therefore this section focuses on both the normal and the abnormal pregnancy in relation to the fluid and electrolyte changes that occur during adulthood.

Pregnancy

Pregnancy is a normal, healthy state accompanied by great changes in fluid and electrolytes that are nevertheless normal for pregnancy and well handled by the woman. For many years these alterations were considered pathophysiologic rather than adaptive, and many persons believed that the pregnant state set the stage for deviations leading to disease. In particular, preeclampsia and eclampsia were thought of as extensions of normal fluid and electrolyte changes and as likely occurrences in "high risk" pregnant women. This philosophy extended to the belief that all pregnant women should be treated with low-sodium diets and diuretic therapy. We have since learned that such therapy probably is much more detrimental than beneficial. Much evidence indicates that preeclampsia is a pathologic state separate from the normal fluid and electrolyte changes during pregnancy and that in reality it is not an exaggeration of these normal changes at all but may be characterized by alterations in the opposite direction. Before the pathophysiology of preeclampsia or eclampsia is described, the physiologic fluid and electrolyte adaptations during normal pregnancy will be discussed in detail.

Hormones of pregnancy. The two major hormones of pregnancy are progesterone and estrogen. They are present in high concentrations throughout pregnancy, although their ratio does change, with proportionately more progesterone being secreted as gestation draws to an end.

Table 11-7. Effects of estrogen and progesterone on fluid, electrolyte, and acid-base balance

Estrogen	Progesterone
Stimulates hepatic synthesis of angiotensinogen Increases water content of skin	Inhibits aldosterone Only weakly able to affect sodium reabsorption (therefore is natriuretic) Increases respiratory drive, causing respiratory alkalosis Decreases HCO_3^- reabsorption

The physiologic effects of these hormones on fluid and electrolyte balance during pregnancy are indicated in Table 11-7. An apparently major effect of the high hormonal levels during pregnancy is the blocking of aldosterone by progesterone at the renal distal convoluted tubule (DCT). You will recall that facilitory sodium reabsorption occurs through the action of aldosterone. Presumably there are hormone receptor sites on the luminal cell membranes in the DCT to which aldosterone normally binds, an occurrence that must necessarily precede any further effects of the hormone on sodium reabsorption. When large concentrations of progesterone are present, less aldosterone is able to bind to the receptor. The stereochemistry of progesterone in some way mimics that of aldosterone. Although it is known that progesterone affects sodium reabsorption, the degree to which this occurs is much less than with aldosterone. Thus the overall result of the competitive binding inhibition of aldosterone by progesterone is natriuretic (i.e., salt wasting). Excessive sodium is lost through the urine, and an overall reduction in body and ECF sodium occurs. Therefore the pregnant state is actually characterized by mild hyponatremia.

Another hormonal effect of possible importance in pregnancy is the stimulation of liver production of a renin substrate, angiotensinogen. This substance may lead to excessive production of angiotensin, a substance that is extraordinarily difficult to measure in the blood. If such a phenomenon did occur, the pressor effects of angiotensin might contribute to blood pressure elevation during pregnancy. However, there is evidence that pregnant women adapt to the high levels of angiotensin. Angiotensin levels are presumed to be high as the result of greatly increased renin levels in pregnancy as well. There is evidence, however, that in normal pregnancy women become adapted to these high levels and, if administered exogenous angiotensin, would require much higher doses to elicit a blood pressure elevation response. The tolerance of the normal pregnant woman to angiotenson does not characterize the pre-eclamptic state.

Renal function. During pregnancy there is an expansion of the TBW, the ECF particularly, and for several other reasons as well the kidneys are required to increase their work to maintain the steady state. A major effect of pregnancy on kidney function is increased RBF and GFR. These increases are most apparent in the early part of pregnancy, with some studies showing evidence of decreases toward normal values in the last trimester. However, there is evidence that many of the studies that documented drops in RBF and GFR were done on pregnant women in the supine position, which creates an important artifact. If a subject lies on her side, it has been shown that the RBF and GFR increase dramatically. There is as much as a 50% increase in RBF, and some studies show increases of the GFR to 300 ml/min. This increased GFR causes an increased work load on the kidneys, since the reabsorption mechanisms of the tubules are then required to transport much more solute than normal. It seems that the capacity to reabsorb becomes overwhelmed in even the normal pregnancy, thus perhaps accounting for the diuresis of pregnancy, as well as the wasting of salt, glucose, and amino acids. The glycosuria of pregnancy is mild but nevertheless is present in the majority of cases. It would not appear that the tubular maximum (T_m) for glucose is changed, but rather that the capacity to transport in a given unit of time is depressed in pregnancy. This proclivity is more marked in women who have a less than normal ability to reabsorb glucose in the nonpregnant state, which theoretically could be the result of previous renal damage caused by minor infections during childhood. The GFR increase in pregnancy not only presents the tubules with greater reabsorption work. A secondary effect appears to be diuresis of dilute urine. Thus the nocturia and frequency experienced so often in early pregnancy, and usually attributed to pressure effects of the growing uterus, may in fact be more physiologic than mechanical.

The cause of the increased RBF and GFR is unknown at this time. One factor is probably the increased ECF that occurs in pregnancy, causing expansion of the plasma volume to values of 30% to 50% over normal by the thirty-fourth week of gestation. This would necessarily result in increased cardiac output (and work load) because of increases in both the heart rate and the stroke volume. Since systolic arterial blood pressure does not change significantly during the normal pregnancy, and since diastolic pressure drops 10 to 15 mm Hg, it is apparent that the peripheral vasculature adapts to the increased volume of blood by arteriolar relaxation. Thus the systolic pressure of the blood does not change with the increasing flow, since total peripheral resistance drops. Renal hemodynamics are altered by this phenomenon because vasodilation of renal arterioles results in augmentation of the RBF and GFR. The relaxation of renal arterioles could be even more pronounced than in other tissue beds. The cause of the arteriolar relaxation is unknown, although progesterone is implicated because it may act to decrease vascular smooth muscle tone.

Additional problems with which the kidneys may have to cope during pregnancy are related to gravitational effects. Pressure of the growing fetus on urinary tract structures may result in stagnation of urine, resulting in colonization of the urine with bacteria and perhaps eventual bacteriuria. In most women this condition is not associated with the typical symptoms of urinary tract infection (burning, urgency, dysuria, nocturia). The bacteria may reproduce in significant enough numbers, however, to produce clinical symptoms, and in either case the threat of pyelonephritis is present. The pathophysiology of pyelonephritis usually involves ascending infection from the urethra to the bladder and thence through the ureters to the kidneys. During pregnancy the ureteral smooth muscle has decreased tone, probably as a result of the high progesterone levels. This decreased muscle tone will cause dilation of the ureters, as well as diminished ureteral peristalsis, both of which may contribute to ascension of bacteria from the bladder. Thus the pregnancy period is marked by an increased probability of urinary tract infection.

The activity of the mother and her general health during pregnancy will also affect renal function. It has been shown that the supine position, which may be assumed with increasing frequency during the latter trimester of pregnancy because of fatigue and general discomfort, will cause compression of the inferior vena cava. Even standing will compress veins during the latter part of pregnancy, although the effect is more pronounced in the supine position. The uterus exerts pressure against the walls of the easily collapsible veins, leading to pooling of blood in the veins of the legs, increased filtration out of the capillaries, and dependent edema. Furthermore, there will be a drop in cardiac output as the venous return decreases. The kidneys will receive less blood than normal, since sympathetic vasoconstriction is the predominant response to the previously mentioned cardiovascular effects. The overall result in terms of renal function is oliguria and decreased sodium, water, and chloride excretion, and it provides nurses with the rationale to encourage some exercise even in later pregnancy for clients who do not have cardiac or pulmonary disease. The exercise should not be sufficient to provoke a great oxygen debt, unless the woman is a conditioned athlete. Mild or moderate exercise is probably beneficial for all healthy pregnant women throughout pregnancy if the individual woman determines the degree of exercise permissible according to heart rate, respiratory rate, and general fatigue. Nurses should therefore spend considerable time with their pregnant clients in assessing cardiovascular, pulmonary, and fluid and electrolyte balance and creating an exercise program with the client that the client will be able to understand and monitor effectively. The left lateral recumbent position should also be recommended for resting.

Fluids and electrolytes during pregnancy. The following statements summarize the changes observed in normal pregnancy. There is an expanded ECF, a decrease in serum sodium, and a drop in serum osmolarity. Hypoalbuminemia, which causes less albumin to be available to bind with many plasma constituents (calcium, magnesium, drugs, hormones), also develops. In general, all the plasma ions except chloride are decreased during pregnancy. Chloride levels are probably increased in compensation for the bicarbonate drop caused by excessive bicarbonate excretion in response to respiratory alkalosis. Potassium deficiency is usually not significant.

TBW, red blood cell mass, plasma volume, and blood volume gradually increase during pregnancy. The TBW increase consists of the water of the fetus, amniotic fluid, and placenta, as well as the increased extracellular volume of the mother, a total of 6.3 liters of water gain. The increased blood volume is due to increases in both the red blood cell mass and the plasma volume. There is stimulation of erythropoiesis, but proportionately more plasma is retained than red cells; thus most pregnant women have decreased hematocrit and hemoglobin values, a situation that is not pathophysiologic. The increased blood volume becomes manifest by the twelfth week of gestation, with an increase of as much as 40% developing by the last weeks of the pregnancy. The blood should theoretically be less viscous than normal because of the decreased hematocrit value and the increased plasma water, which should therefore aid in placental perfusion. However, this phenomenon has not been shown to actually occur.

The retention of water exceeds that of sodium because of the natriuretic effect of progesterone and an increase in the secretion of ADH. Other hormones may also play a role, including prostaglandins, growth hormone, adrenocorticotropic hormone (ACTH), and the "third factor," which is an as-yet-unidentified hormone speculated to cause natriuresis. Because of the increase in plasma water, there is a decrease in plasma osmolarity, which will favor filtration over reabsorption at the capillary level and promote interstitial edema. The latter is a nearly universal occurrence during normal pregnancies, is usually mild, but can become dependent and pitting in about 30% of pregnancies. Of course, dependent edema of the lower extremities is further favored by the venous compression caused by the pregnant uterus. The venous pressure in the femoral veins, for example, may increase by a factor of 10 or more. When the woman lies down at night, the gravitational effects are less severe, and an increased volume of ECF is mobilized. This will result in an increase in RBF and GFR and consequently an increase in urine output during the night (nocturia).

Acid-base balance during pregnancy. The major effect on acid-base balance during pregnancy is related to the alveolar hyperventilation that is characteristic. This is due to increased respiratory drive through the direct stimulation of the neural respiratory centers by progesterone, resulting in an overall increased respiratory burden. The increased cardiac output and limited tolerance to exercise result in shortness of breath, which is most marked in the first trimester and may even be present during rest. The effect of hyperventilation is a drop in the arterial and alveolar P_{CO_2}. The average value for Pa_{CO_2} during pregnancy is 30 mm Hg (normal 40 mm Hg). The compensatory response to the lowered Pa_{CO_2}, which would ultimately cause the pH of the blood to rise, is decreased renal HCO_3^- reabsorption. This causes an equilibrium shift toward the formation of H^+ from carbonic acid dissociation, thus returning the pH to normal values. In the normal pregnancy the woman is able to fully compensate for the respiratory alkalosis; thus the arterial pH is unaffected.

One additional acid-base problem that may arise in early pregnancy is caused by the excessive vomiting that some women suffer as "morning sickness." In early pregnancy many women have a drop in stomach acidity because of decreased production of hydrochloric acid by the gastric mucosa. Thus vomiting at this time does not usually result in hypochloremic alkalosis, as one would ordinarily expect. Later in the pregnancy, stomach pH returns to normal, but by this time the morning sickness has usually stopped. Thus the net effects of vomiting during the first trimester are dehydration and an overall loss of electrolytes.

Acid-base balance can again be disrupted during labor and delivery. A tendency toward metabolic acidosis predominates because of the increased muscular work, the resultant oxygen debt that accumulates, and the consequent lactic acid production that occurs. Furthermore, there may be sedative effects of anesthetics on respiratory compensations for the metabolic acidosis. Another consideration is that most women during labor are not partaking of any calories and therefore are usually ketotic, which will further contribute to the metabolic acidosis.

Preeclampsia. Preeclampsia is the name given to a syndrome consisting of symptoms that develop before the actual state of eclampsia (formerly called toxemia) of pregnancy is manifested. The cause of preeclampsia is not well delineated, but there is undoubtedly a population "at risk." It consists of women experiencing their first pregnancy, very young women, and women carrying a multiple pregnancy. The syndrome consists of generalized edema, proteinuria, and hypertension. It can proceed to eclampsia, which is marked by massive edema, renal failure, severe and uncontrollable hypertension, and convulsions. Death may occur if the problems are not adequately treated, and death of the fetus at this stage is also very likely. The classification of preeclampsia is mild or severe (Table 11-8). The severely preeclamptic woman is considered "toxemic," or eclamptic, if she has a convulsion. This occurs in only about 5% of pregnant women with preeclampsia.

The nurse may play an important role in the detection of preeclampsia, since many of the early signs and symptoms may be ignored by the pregnant woman or considered just part of pregnancy. Careful assessment and complete history taking are therefore essential, since the first complaint may be a mild headache, which on further assessment may be revealed to be accompanied by hypertension and proteinuria. The vast majority of women developing preeclampsia are from the lower socioeconomic groups, especially those without good medical and obstetric care.

The pathophysiology of preeclampsia appears to proceed initially from a renal vascular aberration. However, it is possible that the renal pathol-

Table 11-8. Characteristics of preeclampsia

	Mild	Severe
Edema	Generalized	Massive, generalized with pulmonary edema
Blood pressure	Range of 140/90 to 170/110	Greater than 170/110
Urine output	Greater than 500 ml/24 hr	Less than 500 ml/24 hr
Proteinuria	Less than 5 gm/24 hr	More than 5 gm/24 hr

ogy results from the preeclamptic process itself. The lesion is glomerular and involves swelling of the glomerular endothelial cells. This causes the glomerular capillary lumen to be reduced in size, which in turn impedes GFR and RBF. These values are decreased in preeclampsia, although normally elevated in pregnancy, as previously discussed. There is also some evidence that tubular reabsorptive capacity is decreased as well, with the net effect of oliguria and the production of urine of high specific gravity. Renal failure may eventually occur if the disease progresses.

Not only are the renal vessels involved in preeclampsia and eclampsia, but uterine, retinal, and systemic arterioles are all subject to the swelling and vascular spasms observed in renal arterioles. Thus vision, uterine blood flow, and peripheral resistance are all greatly affected by the progression of the disease. In fact, in preeclampsia the blood flow to all organs is decreased, even when blood volume itself is not changed. The vasospasms decrease perfusion to vital organs and increase the total peripheral resistance. Hypertension of increasingly higher values is the end result if treatment is not carried out. The hypertension may be so severe that a cerebrovascular accident is possible, threatening the mother's life.

Edema is another major characteristic of preeclampsia, and again the cause of the excessive accumulation of fluid is not known. Generally speaking, the edema accumulates quickly and excessively, beyond the normal edema of pregnancy. A rapid weight gain of 2.25 kg (5 lb) or more is therefore an important indicator, along with the other clinical signs and symptoms.

The edema can be very severe and life threatening, causing massive fluid accumulation and pulmonary and cerebral edema. The latter is believed to cause the convulsions, behavioral changes, and coma of the truly eclamptic woman. Hypoxia of the brain caused by vasospasm further contributes to the neurologic symptoms. The interstitial edema contributes to expansion of the ECF, but the plasma volume itself is decreased. The loss of plasma into the interstitial space causes hemoconcentration and increased blood viscosity. This effect further perpetuates microcirculatory stasis, hypoxia, and thrombus formation.

The proteinuria of preeclampsia is most likely related to an increase in glomerular membrane permeability, in which large protein molecules such as albumin leak into the tubular filtrate and, because of their size, cannot be reabsorbed by the limited protein reabsorption mechanisms of the tubular cells. The proteinuria augments the normal state of hypoalbuminemia in pregnancy, which in turn can perpetuate the edema of

Table 11-9. Physical assessment of the preeclamptic patient

	HEENT	Cardiac system	Respiratory system	Fetal system	Renal system	Gastrointestinal system	Neuromuscular system
Inspection	Ophthalmoscopic examination of retina shows AV nicking, ↑ venous-arteriolar diameter, arteriolar spasm, retinal edema, blurred vision, blindness		Dyspnea Hemoptysis	Abruptio placentae Fetal death	↓ Urine output ↑ Specific gravity	Vomiting	Decreased awareness Local twitching Convulsions Headache
Palpation	Facial edema			Uterine contractions	Pitting edema Anasarca	Epigastric pain	
Percussion			Decreased resonance				
Auscultation		Blood pressure: 140/90	Rales Rhonchi Coughing	Loss of fetal heart tones			Deep tendon reflexes: 3+-4+

preeclampsia. Liver hypoxia and damage may also contribute to the lowered plasma proteins.

Electrolyte changes in preeclampsia are not significant, unless, of course, the patient has convulsions, a situation resulting in both respiratory and metabolic acidosis. The overall concentration of sodium is increased, presumably through increased sodium reabsorption. There appears to be an underlying defect in the ability of the preeclamptic, as compared to the normal, pregnant woman to regulate excessive dietary salt intake. The net effect is sodium retention. It is important, however, to realize that salt restriction plays a role only in preeclampsia, not in normal pregnancy. Furthermore, the use of diuretics and salt-poor diets as part of routine obstetric care for all women is meaningless, since it has not been shown to prevent ecclampsia but only to treat the pathology when it is present. There are also many authorities who do not advocate salt-losing diuretics in preeclampsia, since the effects may be more detrimental than positive.

Treatment of the preeclamptic patient is therefore as controversial as the numerous theories of the disease etiology. The major approach, if possible, is to terminate the pregnancy and save both the mother and a viable infant. Preeclampsia does not persist if the pregnancy is no longer present. Other approaches are aimed at preventing the serious complications of the disease, which may involve the kidneys, liver, and heart. Treatment should be carried out in a hospital, and nurses caring for such patients should be well equipped to do complete patient assessment. Nursing care must be based on a thorough understanding of the pathophysiologic progression of this disease. The major areas of treatment are (1) water and electrolyte balance, (2) control of hypertension, and (3) maintenance and normal neurologic status.

Table 11-9 lists the approaches used in the physical assessment of the preeclamptic patient.

CASE STUDY • WOMAN WITH PREECLAMPSIA

IDENTIFYING DATA

Mrs. C. J., a 31-year-old white primigravida, was admitted 1/17. Her last menstrual period was 5/24. She is at approximately 34 weeks' gestation, with an estimated date of confinement (EDC) of 2/21. She has been treated for preeclampsia in an outlying hospital since 12/14.

PERTINENT HISTORY

Client gives history of increased edema since approximately 5 months' gestation. She was hospitalized on 12/14 because of excessive weight gain in the range of 4.5 kg (10 lb) over the previous 2 days. Physical findings at this time included increasing dependent edema and some edema of hands and face, blood pressure elevated to 140/90, and proteinuria of 2+. She gave a history of occasional nonsevere headaches and of sometimes seeing spots in front of her eyes. During her hospitalization she was treated with diuretic therapy, which resulted in mobilization of her edema fluid and a weight loss of approximately 7.2 kg (16 lb). [Diuretic therapy is not always recommended treatment for preeclampsia—see text.] She was also treated with antihypertensive drugs and was receiving hydralazine (Apresoline), 25 mg four times a day, at the time of her admission to the outlying hospital.

Initial creatinine clearance at the time of hospitalization was 97 (70 to 110 ml/min); by 1/14 creatinine clearance had dropped 61 ml/min. The 24-hour urine clearance of protein increased during this time from between 0.33 and 0.61 gm to 1.218 gm. On 1/7 the client was transferred to this hospital for further management of preeclampsia.

LABORATORY DATA

Admission blood counts revealed RBC of 3.53 (3.8 to 6.2/cμmm), hemoglobin level of 12.1 (12 to 16 gm/dl), and hematocrit value of 35.1% (38% to 47%). A blood bicarbonate value of 20 (22-31 mEq/liter), calcium of 7.6 (8.5 to 10.5 mg/dl), and chloride of 111 (95 to 100 mEq/liter) reflected alkalosis. Although serum creatinine remained within normal limits at 1.0 (0.6 to 1.6 mg/dl), the BUN level was 22 (5 to 25 mg/dl). Total serum protein of 4.8 (6.0 to 8.5 gm/dl) reflected the protein loss via the compromised glomeruli. Urine values related to the renal dysfunction included albumin 4+ and 0-1 hyaline casts. A 24-hour urine specimen collected between 1/17 and 1/18 showed a creatinine clearance of 66.5 (70 to 120 ml/min) and a protein level of 1.2 gm (<100 mg). Urine specific gravity was 1.013. All other values were within normal limits with the exception of an alkaline phosphatase value of 220 (30 to 115 mM/ml) and a lactic dehydrogenase (LDH) value of 345 (100 to 250 mM/ml), resulting from the placental and liver deterioration commonly seen in preeclampsia.

PHYSICAL EXAMINATION

General: blood pressure in supine position, 150/100; left lateral position, 150/94; temperature, 36.8° C (98.3° F); pulse rate, 76; respirations, 20; weight, 66.2 kg (147 lb)

HEENT: normocephalic; pupils equal, round, reactive to light and accommodation (PERRLA); fundi benign, no arteriospasms; neck supple; no adenopathy

Lungs: clear

Heart: normal, regular rhythm without murmur or gallops

Abdomen: gravid fundal height, 31 cm; fetal heart rate, 156 beats/min; no hepatosplenomegaly

Extremities: edema of hands and face; no cyanosis

Neurologic study: deep tendon reflex, 3+.

Impression: intrauterine pregnancy at 34 weeks; mild preeclampsia

HOSPITAL COURSE

Initial management of Mrs. C. J. included high-protein diet, bed rest with bathroom privileges, left lateral recumbent position encouraged, hydralazine (Apresoline), 25 mg four times a day, and phenobarbital, 60 mg four times a day. Blood pressure and weight continued to increase despite therapy. On 1/20 urine specific gravity rose to 1.029, as compared with an admission value of 1.013. On the morning of 1/21 blood pressure was 150/108, and a weight gain of 25 kg (5½ lb) had occurred in 24 hours. Amniocentesis revealed an L/S ratio of less than 2, indicating fetal immaturity. In an attempt to expand plasma volume, Mrs. C. J. received 1000 ml D_5LR over 2½ hours. Blood pressure stabilized at 140/90, and the decision was made to defer cesarean section. At 6 P.M. on the evening of 1/21 an additional weight gain of 3.6 kg (8 lb) was recorded. Blood pressure of 152/100, urine protein of 3+, deep tendon reflex of 3 to 4+, complaint of severe headache, and decreased urinary output resulted in transfer to the labor and delivery unit, where Mrs. C. J. was closely monitored. Blood pressure decreased somewhat through the night, but urinary output was drastically reduced, at times dropping to 5 ml/hr, and complaints of severe headache continued. In light of this progressive deterioration the decision was made to terminate the pregnancy via cesarean section. Between 7:30 and 8 A.M. a loading dose of 4 gm of magnesium sulfate was administered and continued at a rate of 2 gm/hr. Estimated blood loss was 1100 ml, and approximately 2000 ml of ECF in the form of ascites was drained off.

Baby Girl J., weighing 1400 gm (3lb 4 oz), was delivered at 9:35 A.M.; Apgar scores were 5 and 7. She was cyanotic and floppy; intubation yielded an immediate response in heart rate. Sodium bicarbonate was administered at the time of resuscitation. Blood-gas determinations taken under 58% O_2 were pH 7.32, PCO_2 18.5, and PO_2 155. Lungs were mostly clear with few rales. There was no retraction or grunting. Admission impression: 34 or 35 weeks, small for gestational age. The evening of admission the infant was started on nasogastric feeding. By 1/23 she was stable and no longer receiving O_2. On 1/30, the day of Mrs. C. J.'s discharge, Baby Girl J. weighed 1490 gms (3lb 14 oz). Her condition was sufficiently stable to permit transfer to the community hospital close to her parents' residence.

After delivery Mrs. C. J.'s blood pressure was 142/90. Throughout the following 24 hours magnesium sulfate was administered at the rate of 1 gm/hr. Blood pressure remained stable, with diastolic pressure not exceeding 86 mm Hg. Urine protein dropped to negative-trace range, but hourly output remained low at 26 to 28 ml. After discontinuation of the magnesium sulfate and transfer to the postpartum unit, Mrs. C. J.'s blood pressure rose briefly. From 8 P.M. until the time of discharge, however, diastolic pressure never exceeded 90 mm Hg, and a general pattern of decreasing systolic and distolic values was seen. Average hourly output steadily rose, with diuresis beginning during the second postoperative day. Urine protein measurements were never higher than 2+. Twenty-four-hour urine collected between 1/27 and 1/28 showed that creatinine clearance had risen to a normal level of 97.2 ml/min. Edema steadily decreased; weight on the fourth postpartum day showed a loss of 7 kg (15 lb 12 oz) since the time of surgery. By 1/28, the fifth postpartum day, bicarbonate levels had risen to a normal value of 23 mEq/liter, BUN levels had fallen to 11 mg/dl, and total protein had risen to 5.2 gm/dl. Hemoglobin and hematocrit values were 9.4 gm/dl and 28.5%, reflecting the 1200 ml blood loss during cesarean section. By the day of discharge an additional weight loss of 6.5 kg (14 lb 8 oz) was recorded, blood pressure was 134/90, and there was a trace of urine protein.

NURSING STRATEGIES

1. Decrease risk of convulsion via accurate monitoring of client status.*
   a. Blood pressure measurement every 4 hours (except between midnight and morning)
   b. Daily weight measurement at same time each day
   c. Daily urine specimen for protein determination
   d. Observation for signs of deterioration, including headache, visual disturbances, epigastric pain, edema, and decreased urinary output
2. Promote stabilization of condition before delivery.
   a. Use of nursing measures to promote intake of high protein diet
   b. Intake of fluid as client desires
   c. Maintenance of bed rest facilitated in left lateral recumbent position
   d. SNS stimulation minimized by providing a dim, quiet environment, with visitors restricted to one at a time†
   e. Explanation and reassurance of client and significant others regarding a sedentary, restrictive regimen for a client who may not look or feel "sick"
3. Prevent iatrogenic effects of pharmacologic therapy.
   a. Magnesium sulfate to effectively reduce the risk of convulsion via blocking transmission at the myoneural junction, decreasing muscle fiber excitability, and depressing the CNS (The hazard of magnesium sulfate toxicity is very real, however, since this drug is excreted via the kidney. Therefore it is not administered unless patellar reflex can be elicited, urinary output has been

---

*Frequency of various measurements should be increased as client's condition warrants and supplemented by checks of deep tendon reflexes and frequent evaluation of 24-hour urine creatinine clearance and protein levels.
†Telephone and television may be restricted as condition requires, although judicious use of television may have a relaxing effect on some clients.

100 ml or more in previous 4 hours, and respiratory rate exceeds 12 to 14/min.)
  b. Hydralazine a valuable antihypertensive agent because it mediates decreased arteriolar resistance via vasodilation (The risk of decreased uteroplacental perfusion stems from a precipitous drop in blood pressure, thus the aim of therapy is to stabilize diastolic pressure near 90 to 100 mm Hg.)
  4. Deliver surviving child via accurate monitoring of fetal status.
    a. Daily observation of fetal heart rate; more frequent observation if condition deteriorates
    b. Evaluation of various means of assessing fetal status, including stress and nonstress tests, amniocentesis for L/S ratio, and hormone levels in blood and urine

DISCHARGE PLANNING

A client who is adequately prepared for discharge will understand the importance of follow-up evaluation to rule out permanent renal or cardiovascular dysfunction. She should be evaluated within 2 weeks after leaving the hospital and again at 6 weeks postpartum. By this time all hypertension and proteinuria should have abated.

Reduced activity levels should be maintained until renal and cardiovascular status has returned to normal. If the infant's condition permits discharge home, the parents should be helped to plan for assistance with child care so that the mother has adequate rest periods.

A period of at least 12 months should elapse before the next pregnancy, to permit restoration of compromised body tissues and replenishment of nutritional stores. If blood pressure returns to normal within the postpartum period, oral contraceptives are not contraindicated should the client prefer them. An alternative method of conception control will be necessary for the 6 weeks before documentation of a normotensive state and for 6 weeks after the initiation of an oral contraceptive regimen, until ovulation is safely suppressed.

SENESCENCE

A pattern of changes in fluid, electrolyte, and acid-base balance occurs throughout the senescent process, which begins to be manifested from the age of about 30 years onward. These alterations in balance lead to predispositions of the elderly to imbalances, and an understanding of both the physiology of senescence and the common disorders of senescence is necessary for nurses to give rational, intelligent nursing care. Aging involves every system of the body and is characterized by decrements in all physiologic functions and in the ability to maintain the steady state when the normal function is disrupted by pathosis. Although aging is a universal, irrevocable phenomenon, the rate of aging is nevertheless determined by certain individual characteristics, within limits. It is incorrect to dogmatically state that a change in function is present in all individuals over the age of 70 years, and it is equally incorrect for the nurse planning care for an elderly client to make similar assumptions. Cognizance of these individual differences will highlight the importance of nursing assessment of every client, with regard to all physiologic or pathophysiologic states.

General characteristics

Some of the most obvious changes that occur with aging are those of body size and shape. With advancing age there is increasing weight, which, after about 70 years of age, is not statistically apparent, but this may be due only to the effect of obesity on morbidity. The excess weight that collects is largely adipose tissue. The result is an overall decrease in total body density with age. Furthermore, one effect of increasing adiposity is decreased TBW. Although the plasma volume and extracellular fluid space do not change significantly with age, there is a decrease in TBW. Within certain structures there is decreased hydration as well; thus there is a differential effect of aging on certain tissues and organs. The major tissue affected by senescence is connective tissue. There is increasing rigidity of connective tissue with aging because of a decreasing ratio of hexosamine to collagen, and a cross linking of collagen molecules occurs, binding tissue into a less flexible structural framework. Connective tissue is largely structural in its action, giving form to vessels, binding organs together, forming capsules for organs, and of course providing support for the body as bones and cartilage. As the density of connective tissue increases, its function becomes increasingly impaired. Thus many of the changes that occur with aging are secondary to connective tissue changes. For example, arteriosclerosis is a universal phenomenon with aging, and it will affect the oxygenation and nutrition of most tissues if it progresses. The pathogenesis of arteriosclerosis involves collagen changes in the arteriolar walls, imparting greater rigidity to them and thus causing these vessels to offer increased resistance to blood flow. Ultimately the flow to the organs supplied will become impaired. Since the age-related changes in connective tissue are accompanied by decreased hydration of the tissue, less of the TBW is distributed throughout all the connective tissue of the body. The moisture of connective tissue is essential to its normal function, and thus the decreased hydration further perpetuates the decrements in function.

Significant electrolyte changes also occur with aging. Although total body concentrations of sodium and chloride do not appear to be significantly altered, there is a gradual decrease in total body levels of potassium with age. Calcium also changes with aging because of the osteoporotic process that accompanies normal aging. There is less bone calcium and less total body calcium with aging.

Another interesting effect of senescence is the increasing H^+ concentration of the ECF, leading to a drop in pH to a value of about 7.36, which is accompanied by a corresponding increase in P_{CO_2} and decrease in HCO_3^- concentration. This suggests a state of partially compensated respiratory acidosis. As will be discussed, decrements in both respiratory and renal function contribute to this phenomenon.

Renal changes

The size and volume of the kidneys decrease greatly with age after reaching their maximum at the age of 30 to 40 years. The alterations with age are due to a decrease in the number of glomeruli, to a value of about two-thirds the number in the young adult. Furthermore, there are distinct changes in the structure of the glomeruli and nephrons. One alteration is a thickening of the glomerular capillary basement membrane. This change would obviously impede filtration from the blood into Bowman's capsule, decreasing GFR, which definitely decreases dramatically with aging to values as low as 94 ml/min. Other phenomena contribute to the decreased GFR, a primary one being decreased RBF. However, it has also been demonstrated that the drop in RBF matches the loss of nephrons. As glomeruli degenerate, shunting of blood from arterioles to venules occurs, with resultant decreased RBF. It is believed that renal vascular changes occur with age, and as a result the kidneys are subject to increasing hypoxia and ischemia, thus becoming gradually less functional.

There are tubular changes, such as thickening of tubular basement membranes, and dilation and even pouch formation of the collecting ducts. Therefore tubular reabsorption and secretion are interrupted. Some variables that are affected include urea clearance, with a resultant rise in the BUN levels, acidification, which is reduced, and glucose reabsorption, which is decreased because of a drop in the T_m for glucose. The ability of the kidneys to concentrate the urine is markedly decreased in the elderly, with a drop in the maximum specific gravity of the urine of 1.030 to 1.023 in the 90-year-old man. Of course, the implication is that the senescent kidney must increase its output to allow for the excretion of the obligatory metabolic wastes. Yet the kidney in the aged person, with its decreased RBF and GFR, is not always able to accommodate this increased output requirement, since the urine production is decreased from the normal adult value of 1.0 ml/min to 0.8 ml/min in the elderly. The result is a tendency for the aged person to have an increased BUN level and a lesser ability to handle an acid load.

Integumentary changes

The changes that occur in connective tissue with aging have already been mentioned. Since the skin is composed of an epidermis and a dermis, the latter composed mainly of connective tissue, there are remarkable changes in the composition and physiology of the integument. The wrinkling of the skin gives testimony to this fact. With regard to fluid and electrolyte balance, the age-related skin changes are significant. Since the skin is the major thermoregulatory organ, its surface allows for IWL. In the aged person there is a decreased hydration of the skin, which has several effects. An obvious one is the annoying dryness and itching of the skin. The senescent skin is also less able to participate in thermoregulation. Alterations in the evaporative ability of the skin reduce IWL, and there are also atrophic changes in the sweat glands, with a decreased ability to perspire. Furthermore, vascular declines cause a decrease in skin circulation, which will only exacerbate the decreased IWL and sweating problems. All these factors contribute to the inability of the elderly person to handle a heat load such as that produced by fever, hyperthermia, or exercise. For this reason the aged individual is at risk for conditions such as heat stroke. Any measure that nurses can take to increase the circulation to the skin and decrease the dryness and thickness of the skin will help to promote normal fluid balance. The use of massage and lotions and limited exercise to promote activity of the sweat glands all have a place in the nursing care plan.

Cardiac and vascular changes

The heart and blood vessels are profoundly affected with increasing age. Cardiac function declines, and peripheral vascular atherosclerotic thickening results in a decreased ability of the heart to adequately perfuse vital organs. These changes are mentioned in regard to fluid, electrolyte, and acid-base balance because all organs and tissues that participate in the regulation of these various balances may be affected by decreased perfusion, hypoxia, and atrophy. This situation was described for the kidneys particularly, but all organs are involved. Gastrointestinal tract function is disturbed through these senescent declines, and even endocrine function may be affected.

Respiratory changes

The compliance of the lungs and respiratory muscles decreases with age, and there is a reduction in the volume of the thoracic cage because of skeletal changes such as kyphosis and osteoporosis. Furthermore, the pulmonary capillary network may be disrupted by senescent changes. The incidence of emphysematous changes is very high in the elderly. These alterations in anatomy and physiology lead to a susceptibility of the elderly to respiratory tract infections and impairs the ability of the respiratory tract to compensate for metabolic acid-base problems. They also lead to a mild respiratory acidosis in the elderly person, which may be poorly compensated by the decreased acidification functions of the aged kidney. The respiratory changes also limit the ability of the elderly person to exercise, since there are altered ventilation-perfusion ratios, decreased diffusion, and decreased compliance in the lungs.

Gastrointestinal tract changes

Major changes occur with aging in the gastrointestinal tract. Some changes are related to long-standing hypoxia caused by vascular insufficiency, and others are due to atrophy, which is a concomitant of the aging process. Thus the production of hydrochloric acid is frequently decreased, as are other gastrointestinal secretions. In addition, changes in the mucosa impair the transport of fluids, electrolytes, and nutrient molecules across this diffusion barrier. Therefore gastrointestinal function with relation to fluid, electrolyte, or acid-base balance may be considerably diminished.

Implications of senescence

All the previously described alterations in organ structure and function ultimately result in the fragile steady state of the elderly. The presence of degenerative changes as well as pathologic states such as diabetes or heart disease will limit the ability of the aged person to cope with deviations from the normal. Any stressor may be sufficient to completely and irrevocably disrupt the steady state. Fluid losses or gains may be a great problem in terms of homeostasis. An elderly person undergoing surgery not only will be more likely to develop water intoxication but also will be less likely to recover. The same principle applies to almost any disease condition that a very old person might develop, from diarrhea to pneumonia. These considerations must be made an essential part of the nursing care plan for the elderly, whether or not the initial problem is a fluid, electrolyte, or acid-base one. In many cases such problems will develop as the result of another pathosis. No matter what condition the elderly person might have initially, nurses are obligated to adequately and intelligently assess fluid, electrolyte, and acid-base balance, utilizing the developmental considerations discussed in this chapter.

12

Principles of fluid therapy

MARY ELLEN BANKS

The assessment and administration of oral and parenteral fluids, as part of maintenance and replacement therapy for patients with a compromised volume or electrolyte status, are a nursing responsibility. Safe and effective fluid intervention requires a synthesis of concepts relevant to body water and electrolyte dynamics, as well as a clear understanding of human development. In addition, a nurse needs practiced psychomotor skills to administer oral and parenteral fluids to a client, as well as communication skills that guarantee an accurate record of the fluids and electrolytes provided to the individual.

This chapter will (1) describe the essential components of careful client assessment and the equipment and steps used for administration of fluids and electrolytes; (2) outline the necessity, rationale, and procedures for carefully monitoring clients receiving fluid therapy; and (3) show graphic and summative examples of appropriate methods for recording a client's intake and output. The chapter will use developmental guidelines to present content related to providing a client with fluids and electrolytes. Special emphasis will be given to the problems and needs of the infant, child, adolescent, adult, and older adult.

ASSESSMENT AND DATA BASE DETERMINATION

Assessment of the fluid state of an individual should be comprehensive and multidimensional. Such physical observation not only can corroborate clinical laboratory data but also can serve as an ongoing account of the client's condition. Careful assessment is a vital step in fluid administration. Table 12-1 represents such a multidimensional assessment tool.

252

Monitoring the physical state of the client before initiation of treatment provides a baseline for evaluation of the effects of care during fluid and electrolyte administration. Continual assessment of these same functions will demonstrate either return to the normal hydration state or the effects of inappropriate compensation if too little or too much fluid was given to a client. The frequency of such hydration checks is dependent on the severity and acute nature of the illness episode and should be individualized according to the needs of the client. Frequency levels outlined in Table 12-1 are suggestions that may need modification in varying circumstances.

Maintenance requirements for fluids and electrolytes represent the number of milliliters or milliequivalents, respectively, that the body needs each day to match daily losses from these two components. The goal of such balanced therapy is to maintain homeostasis in both wellness and illness. Reference to Tables 11-1 to 11-3 permits calculation of a given person's fluid needs according to weight.

Some persons in illness states require fluids and electrolytes in addition to those needed to maintain homeostasis. These fluids are referred to as replacement fluids, and they represent fluids and electrolytes depleted in excess of normal body losses. Such extraordinary decreases are of major significance and may be caused by nasogastric aspirates and drainage, wound or fistula drainage, ascites, increased body temperature, hemorrhage, or losses ascribed to gastrointestinal malabsorption. The amount and kind of replacement fluid given to an individual patient depend on the estimation of the amount and kind of excess fluid losses.

In wellness states nearly all persons can attain and maintain their own fluid and electrolyte balance. During infancy and childhood the adult caretaker provides the child with needed fluids and liquids. Therefore teaching parents the essential elements of fluid requirements helps to assure that the child will receive the optimal volume of liquids. This teaching is concerned not only with making available to the infant or child the basic amount of liquid but also with how to make modifications based on increased environmental temperature and on illness with increased body temperature and diarrhea.

The older adult may also need assistance in maintaining proper body hydration. The older adult's problems in relation to mobility, the use of diuretics, depression and apathy, financial impingements, oral irregularities, urinary incontinence, and even the care provided by others (which can be abusive or neglectful) can all affect his ability to indepen-

Table 12-1. Physical assessment guide for fluid and electrolyte status

Body area	Pertinent observation	Probable cause or usefulness	Frequency (to be checked and charted)
Weight (percentage of loss expressed as decrease from normal, healthy weight)*	Loss (%): 2-5 6-9 10-14 15 20	Mild dehydration Moderate dehydration Severe dehydration Extreme dehydration Death (usually)	On admission, every 12-24 hr
Foot length (positive correlation between foot and body length and gestational age; indirect method for computing fluid and drug requirements, since foot length is also a correlate of weight)	Foot measured from heel to toes; identification print measured as well during immediate neonatal period	Usefulness: accessible measure for determining fluid requirements, especially when newborn is critically ill	On admission (especially useful with infants when physical condition precludes obtaining weight)
HEENT Fontanel (anterior)	Depressed Full, bulging	Fluid volume deficit Fluid volume overload	Every 1 hr, infants only (measure height or depression)
Eyes	Sunken, dry conjunctiva Absence of tearing	Fluid volume deficit Fluid volume deficit	Every 4 hr
Mouth	Sticky, dry membranes Saliva has increased viscosity	Fluid volume deficit Sodium deficit	Every 2 hr
Tongue	Longitudinal furrows	Sodium deficit	Every 2 hr
Lips	Dry, cracked	Fluid volume deficit	Every 4 hr
Bridge of nose	Pinched skin remains raised	Fluid volume deficit Decreased skin turgor	Every 2 hr
Cheek	Chvostek's sign	Tetany, potassium deficit	Every 4 hr
Cardiopulmonary system Cardiovascular system	Increased pulse rate Decreased pulse rate Pulse quality, bounding Blood pressure, low Changes in percussible heart size or deviation from normal axis Cardiac arrhythmias	Fluid volume deficit Fluid volume deficit Fluid volume overload Fluid volume deficit Fluid volume overload Potassium deficit	Every 1 hr (pulse and blood pressure until stable)

Assessment	Observations	Significance	Frequency
Respiratory system	Breath sounds Rales, rhonchi	Fluid volume overload	Every 1 hr
Gastrointestinal system Abdomen	Hyperperistalsis Pinched skin on lower abdomen remains raised	Diarrheal losses Decreased skin turgor	Every 2 hr
Renal system Kidney-bladder Child-adult catheterization with urinometer and infant-sized catheter or adhesive 24-hr urinary collection bag	Diuresis Decreased kidney output 10 ml/hr	Fluid volume deficit Fluid volume deficit	Every 1 hr
Extremities Dependent body parts Sacrum Back Legs	Edema—represented by increasing degrees of fluid collection (e.g., 1+, 2+, 3+, 4+)	Fluid volume overload Decreased venous return	Every 2 hr
Integumentary system Temperature Generalized skin surfaces	Increased Decreased Cold, decreased turgor Cold, clammy, decreased turgor Warm or cold, turgor normal, doughy feeling Dry, scaly skin, dry mucous membranes, including female genitalia Velvety sheen	Sodium excess Fluid volume deficit Isotonic dehydration Hypotonic dehydration Sodium deficit Hypertonic dehydration Sodium excess Fluid volume deficit	Every 1 hr
Neurologic status	Apathetic, hypotonic, coma, restlessness, hyperirritability, convulsions	Hypernatremia Fluid volume deficit Fluid volume overload	Every 30 min

*Fluid requirements for wellness and illness states are based on the respective weights for those states.

dently achieve and maintain water and electrolyte balance. One of these problems or an operative combination of them can place the older adult at serious risk for both fluid and electrolyte imbalance. This can be especially evident in the older client who is seeking emergency hospitalization for an acute illness or an accident, since it is often necessary to delay treatment until fluid and electrolyte homeostasis can be achieved. Delaying treatment for such a reason may be an additional stressor to the client, who may already be confused and upset because of the need to be hospitalized.

ORAL MAINTENANCE AND REPLACEMENT

Liquids and the water content of solid foods provide the fluids required in the wellness state. Even during illness, oral administration of fluid and electrolytes is appropriate as long as the person is alert, is not vomiting, is not having profound fluid loss, and does not have a mechanical obstruction of the alimentary tract. Even if a regular diet cannot be tolerated, the use of fluids may still be suitable, and selection should be governed by the limitations of the illness and the preferences of the client.

A discussion of oral maintenance and replacement therapy should consider the mild forms of acute illness when infants, children, or adults with such conditions as viral diarrhea, an upper respiratory infection, fever, or other mild illness have potential or actual mild fluid and electrolyte disturbances. The confident home management of such situations before they progress to serious acute states can strengthen the client's or caretaker's coping mechanisms and decrease the chance for more serious illness in the child or adult. In addition, in the hospital setting oral fluids are often used after a person recovers from anesthesia or sedation for surgery or a diagnostic procedure but before solid foods are reintroduced. Thus in these situations hydration of the organism is a consideration as the body's tolerance for feeding is reestablished. Oral fluids that are often suggested for this purpose include water; flattened carbonated beverages such as colas, lemon-lime soda, and ginger ale; unthickened flavored gelatin; Gatorade; and broth. In addition, such commercial formula preparations as glucose in water and oral electrolyte solutions may be recommended. Table 12-2 provides information regarding these products.

The indication for use of any particular fluid varies with the cause of fluid and electrolyte depletion. With diarrhea not only water is lost, but electrolytes are lost as well. In approximately 70% of diarrhea cases there is a proportional loss of fluid and electrolytes, expressed as isotonic de-

Table 12-2. Oral fluids

Solution	Calories (Kcal/30 ml)	HCO₃ (mEq/liter)	Na⁺ (mEq/liter)	Ca⁺⁺ (mEq/liter)	K⁺ (mEq/liter)	Mg⁺⁺ (mEq/liter)	Cl⁻ (mEq/liter)	Predominant carbohydrate
Water								
Pedialyte (oral electrolyte solution)	6.0		30.0	4.0	20.0	4	30.0	Dextrose
Lytren (oral electrolyte solution)	9.0 (isotonic)		30.0	4.0	25.0	4	25.0	Glucose
5% glucose in water	6.0							Glucose
10% glucose in water	12.0							Glucose
Pepsi-Cola	13.2	7.3	6.5		0.8			Sucrose
Coca-Cola	14.4	13.4	0.4		12.0			Sucrose
Ginger ale	10.0	3.6	3.5					Sucrose
Gatorade	5.5		23.0		3.0		17.0	Glucose
Lemon-lime soda	9.6		7.5					Sucrose
Broth, beef (canned)	6.0		55.0	0.3	0.2			
Tea, unsweetened	0.25					Trace		

hydration. In this situation giving a person water or a solution, such as tea, that does not contain electrolytes can lead to continued fluid loss and a concomitant loss of electrolytes, causing hypotonic dehydration. If in this same situation a solution such as undiluted condensed broth is offered to the client, hypernatremia and hypertonic dehydration may develop because the solute load exceeds that normally needed by the individual. Comparing the relative values of the various fluids included in Table 12-2, one can see that the choice of a solution depends on the cause of fluid loss and on which oral fluid will most adequately replace those losses.

Another factor to consider in rehydration in diarrheal states is the type of carbohydrate and amount of calories provided by an oral supplementation. The carbohydrate provision, in the form of glucose, sucrose, or maltose, acts as a catalyst for sodium and water absorption. In addition, the calories, even though fewer than those needed for normal daily body metabolism, diminish the effects of catabolism and help decrease tissue utilization. Caution must be used in the selection of carbohydrate for rehydration because absorption of carbohydrate may be impaired during an acute diarrheal episode. One study (Nichols and associates, 1973) demonstrating an osmolar gap between stool osmolality and available osmoles found large quantities of lactate and organic acids present in the feces. It could be generalized (Ford and Haworth, 1963) that the production of such by-products is due to the action of gut flora on undigested carbohydrates and that this process potentially aggravates metabolic acidosis. Therefore complex carbohydrates such as lactose might exacerbate a diarrheal state if such products are reintroduced too soon, or inclusion of lactose in the diet during the acute diarrheal phase would increase the untoward effects of the process.

In acute illness characterized by increased body temperature, in which there is commonly a 10% increase in metabolic demands for each degree of temperature above normal, or in hypernea, in which both caloric and fluid needs are increased, supplementing the child or adult with fluids high in carbohydrates will assist in meeting caloric intake and will decrease untoward effects of the catabolic process. In respiratory disorders with the potential for respiratory acidosis, offering a person an oral supplement high in calories can have a positive compensatory effect. Oral preparations such as Gatorade, specifically devised to replace electrolytes lost through increased sweating from physical exertion, may be appropriate to the febrile state, or they could be offered to infants, children, or debilitated adults when the environmental temperature is increased, especially when air-conditioned areas are unavailable for client use. Oral electrolyte preparations such as Pedialyte and Lytren are available in drug and grocery stores and do not need a physician's prescription for use. Such preparations, as judged by their composition, would provide the most physiologically appropriate supplementation and thus the safest means of rehydration for mild diarrhea, not only for the infant at home, but for the hospitalized infant as well. These solutions would be efficacious for clients who are being withdrawn from intravenous therapy as oral feedings are reintroduced. Carbonated beverages can also be effectively used with diarrheal states when metabolic acidosis is present, since a beverage such as Coca-Cola replaces the decreased bicarbonate reserves.

Developmental considerations in oral fluid administration

The administration of fluids to a client either by mouth or by nasogastric or nasojejunal tube is regulated by the developmental accomplishments and cognitive level of the particular individual. In the young child regressive behavior may need to be recognized and acknowledged so that proper hydration can be achieved. For example, the acutely ill 16-month-old infant who has recently surrendered the bottle may revert to nipple feeding during a period of illness and stress. Since hydration is vital, such a regression is actually a desirable retreat to an earlier stage. After the illness episode, the child who has been supported at the optimal level of functioning during a crisis will return to previously acquired stages of independence that are developmentally and chronologically appropriate.

With children as well as adults, maintaining as much independence and control as possible, as well as providing choices if suitable, helps promote a return to optimal hydration. Calculation of the allowable volume of fluids for a 24-hour period permits mutual goal setting with the parents, client, or other participants in caregiving in regard to the amounts of fluid to be provided at intervals throughout the day. The choice of utensils used to administer fluids may yield fuller cooperation of the client for meeting daily fluid needs. Table 12-3 summarizes devices that may prove useful to the nurse for administering fluids herself or for teaching other caregivers ways to facilitate fluid administration.

Table 12-3. Utensils for providing oral fluids

Utensil	Need	Rationale	Nursing advantages	Nursing problems or concerns
Nasogastric tube	Oral cavity or upper alimentary barrier Comatose patient Decreased suck reflex Decreased gag reflex	Allows for careful attention to complete dietary needs of client receiving tube feedings to prevent hydration and electrolyte deficiencies; same principles regarding oral rehydration applies to client with tube (e.g., infant with Pierre Robin syndrome who develops viral gastroenteritis)	Can control and monitor intake for volume and nutrients	Aspiration Nosocomial infection Increased solute load with carbohydrate (may cause chronic diarrhea) Provision of sucking opportunities for infants Provision of oral hygiene to all clients with tube feedings
Bottle or nipple feeding	Developmentally normal until late infancy or toddlerhood (10-18 mo); may be prolonged in some cultural groups, just as breast feeding may be May be seen in toddlers or even preschoolers if regression during illness includes coping mechanisms of earlier, more secure age; some children with long-standing chronic illness may not have surrendered bottle at this age	Provides sucking experiences that aid in oral musculature development and provide stimulation, pleasure, and relaxation	Can easily monitor intake for volume and nutrients Use of volume-control feeder can provide precise feeding volume (in milliliters)	Nipple size and hardness may make breast-fed baby who needs clear liquids difficult to feed Increased nipple hole size could cause baby to ingest more air, causing increased gastric discomfort

Device	Rationale	Purpose	Nursing considerations
			Crisis not time to make radical changes. Caution regarding allowing infant to sleep with bottle in mouth or propping bottle (important in preventing bottle caries and otitis media, respectively)
Spoon Medicine spoon Medicine cup Regular cup or glass	Use of cup or spoon for assisted or self feeding recognizes developmental accomplishments that foster independence for child and adult with gag and swallow reflex	Use of spoon or small cup to supply client initially with small amounts of liquid or to provide small amounts of fluid at frequent intervals	Proper positioning of client to prevent aspiration. Spilling can occur easily. Sometimes hard to estimate amount of fluids taken. May need to stimulate swallow reflex. Young infants with tongue protrusion have increased tendency to spit out fluids. Place fluids in buccal space. Can be useful technique for coaxing client to drink liquids. School-age children may enjoy saving cups. Preschoolers may be enticed to drink by colors of liquids as viewed through clear-plastic cups. Small cups easy to handle by children or by persons weakened by illness
Syringe or dropper	Use of syringe or dropper recognizes that person has swallow or gag reflex present but may be too weak to drink larger amounts of fluid at one time	To provide individual with controlled measure of fluid and to provide small amounts of fluid at frequent intervals	Fluids safer to administer than from spoon. More accurate monitoring of amount ingested. Spilling not a problem

ADMINISTRATION OF PARENTERAL FLUIDS

The goal of parenteral fluid administration generally is to correct or prevent fluid and electrolyte disturbances in persons who are acutely ill or who may become acutely ill. Specifically, IV fluids may be used to deliver water, electrolytes, and blood components and to serve as a vehicle for medication infusion. Principles related to correct needle placement and infusion techniques are applicable to all clients, regardless of age, who require such treatment. Developmental considerations are paramount in guaranteeing the safety of the client. Innovative equipment has enhanced the maintenance of safety for the individual receiving IV therapy. The human factor not only must emphasize caring and safety but also must minimize error. Familiarity with the technologic aspects of IV therapy helps the client receive the benefits of the best possible care. Not only is IV therapy an expected procedure in the acute care setting, but there is an increasing expectation that nurses in community agencies also have expertise with IV therapy for client management and supervision in home settings.

IV solutions

The various kinds of IV solutions available are formulated to meet client needs matched to the deficits of an acute episode. In addition, IV fluids may be used prophylactically to decrease the chance of dehydration during the presurgical state. For example, the infant or adult at high risk for surgery because of concurrent debilitative states may even have an IV solution started as soon as oral intake is withheld during the 8- to 10-hour fasting period before surgery. If a person is optimally hydrated presurgically, the risks of possible surgical complications such as hemorrhage may be more easily controlled. The IV solutions have different carbohydrate and caloric concentrations, osmolarities, viscosities, pH values, and electrolyte combinations. Table 12-4 reviews some of that information.

Administering an IV solution

Patient cooperation during an invasive procedure can be enhanced by preparing the person for what to expect at various phases of treatment. With children or adults who are to receive IV therapy, gaining their trust and explaining both the short- and long-term goals can reduce fear and allay stress. Developmental considerations are useful in planning IV intervention with children and adults. For example, a child, particularly one who developmentally utilizes fantasy as either a coping mechanism or

Table 12-4. Composition of common IV solutions (mEq/liter)

Solution	Na$^+$	Cl$^-$	K$^+$	Ca^{++}	Mg^{++}	PO$_4$	HCO$_3^-$
0.9% saline	154	154					
Ringer's lactate	130	109	4	3			28
Ionosol D	140	103	10	5	3		55
Ionosol G	63	150	17				
Ionosol T	40	40	35			15	20
Ionosol MB	25	22	20		3	3	
Ionosol DM	80	64	36	5	3		60
Ionosol B	59	52	25		6	13	25

a creative outlet, may view intravenous treatment as one that adults use to control the child by maintaining sedation. In the acutely ill child (or even adult), both the perception and the conscious memory of treatment events may be distorted. The insertion and stabilization of an IV needle may have been one of the few events in which the child was able to energetically participate in his care, and if exhaustion and sleep immediately followed this event, the conclusion that all IV therapy results in sleep might seem logical to the child.

Children might not only fantasize but truly believe and fear that an IV line can also allow their body, blood, or energy to flow out of the tube, as well as let fluids and blood into the body. This belief is not unlike that of the uneasy adult who constantly watches his infusion set because he has misconceptions regarding the potential danger of any kind of air bubble or regarding his fate if the infusion bag or bottle should run dry. Careful explanations and, if necessary, repeated explanations should be part of patient teaching. With children, care must be used to provide information that the child understands. Children may suffer undue stress or anticipatory concern if either too much information or information too far in advance of the events to transpire is provided.

Steps in IV needle placement and stabilization

Equipment selection is synonymous with providing safe IV fluid administration to the patient. Needle size and composition, tubing, in-line filters, drip chambers, and volume control devices are all nursing considerations. In addition, adherence to infection control guidelines, as suggested by the U.S. Center for Disease Control and as interpreted and implemented by hospital infection control committees, also safeguard the patient from infection, the greatest IV therapy hazard.

Basic to any procedure used in a patient's therapy is the principle that the person performing that task have skill and practice with the procedure. Many hospitals have IV infusion teams composed of specially trained nurses whose main function is to initiate and restart IV infusions, including, in some situations, IV cutdowns in a peripheral vein. The rationale for maintaining such a staff is that the hospital then has a group of persons who have demonstrated expertise in an area that will both provide the client with the most expedient care and save time for the other nursing responsibilities. Other hospitals take the stance that all nurses need to have skills of IV therapy initiation, whereas in some teaching hospitals, and particularly on specialty units such as the neonatal or pediatric areas, the house physician and resident staff may assume responsibility for all IV placement. Such issues will have to be managed with concern for the best means of meeting a client's need for rehydration, and will vary at each facility.

An assemblage of equipment needed to insert an IV line and connnect it to a bottle or bag with a solution to be infused includes the following:
1. Arm board
2. Needles and catheters
3. Tourniquet
4. Antiseptic cleaning pads: povidone-iodine (Betadine) or 70% isopropyl alcohol or both
5. IV bottle on stand or bed pole connected with all the appropriate tubing to the junction point where the tubing connects either to the catheter or needle hub

Having all equipment ready expedites the process for the nurse and the client.

Step 1 • Review with the client what you plan to do. Plan with the client or the child's parents the favored sleep positions, hand dominance, and other preferences so that the IV infusion will interfere as little as possible with normal activity. Seek any history of skin sensitivity to tape or cleansing agents.

Step 2 • Examine potential infusion sites. Compare opposing sides. Use of a tourniquet to assess vein distensibility allows the nurse to select an optimal route for infusion.

COMMONLY USED IV SITES

Infant	*Child*	*Adult*	*Older adult*
Scalp	Hands	Hands	Hands
Hands	Arms	Arms	Arms
Feet	Feet		

1. Scalp veins are easily accessible in the young infant, although there may be edema during the first 24 to 48 hours after a vaginal delivery, which makes the site unusable.

2. In the majority of persons the hands have the most readily available superficial veins. Care must be taken to enter the vein at the most distal portion, since it may be necessary to change sites, and the proximal continuation could still be used.

3. In infants the arms are usually not a choice for IV infusion, since the veins are located in the fleshy parts over the muscles and are difficult to enter. The tissue in the child or adult may be leaner, and if hand veins are inaccessible, the use of these veins is permissible. In an older person the veins and surrounding tissue may be very flaccid, and the veins tend to slide or roll when the IV needle is inserted into the skin. In all age groups the use of the antecubital vein is discouraged. Use of this vein as a first choice would make the vein distal to that point unavailable for other infusion sites. The antecubital vein is also the most accessible for obtaining venous blood samples, and use of the site should therefore be retained.

4. It is acceptable to use the feet in infants and children for IV infusion, although this site would be a last option. The feet and lower legs would be contraindicated in most adults, especially elderly persons, because of actual or potential poor venous return. This is especially true if the person has known circulatory problems. Contraindications for using leg or foot veins may even be present in children who are diabetic or have spina bifida.

Step 3 • Remove all extraneous debris. For example, it is necessary to remove blood, mucus, or dead skin before applying a skin disinfectant. Disagreement abounds regarding the necessity of shaving hair. Shaving a portion of an infant's scalp to allow vein visualization and to create space for securing the needle is not questioned, but a problem is evident when the need to shave the hair on an adult's arm is considered. Shaving is believed to disturb the skin's protective function and may cause a local reaction around the IV site. Some practitioners would argue that shaving an IV site should be a matter of individual choice; for instance, if the client is hirsute, taping and retaping the IV site would be uncomfortable.

Practitioner disagreement also is evident regarding the kind of disinfectant to use for skin cleansing. A disinfectant with iodine as the active ingredient is preferable. Such preparations as Betadine have been judged to have a rapid-acting effect and are notable bactericidal, fungicidal, and sporicidal agents. If the patient is known to have an iodine allergy, 70% isopropyl alcohol may be substituted.

Cleanse the area, using outward, circular motions initiated at the proposed point of cannulation. Betadine tints the skin and makes the veins more visually prominent. Once the skin is prepared, it should not be touched again.

Step 4 • To distend the vein, apply the tourniquet proximal to or above the proposed site. Vein distention makes it easier to palpate and visualize the vein. Crying in infants and children results in increased venous pressure and causes vein distention, which facilitates needle insertion. The veins of dark-skinned persons are more difficult to visualize, but the process can be made easier by using a tourniquet for adequate vein distention and by wetting the skin for increased visibility. Other techniques used in conjunction with the aforementioned means of establishing venous distention include wrapping the proposed site with warm compresses to cause venous dilation, tapping the vein to increase blood flow toward the tourniquet, and having the cooperative client clench and unclench his hand so that the action of the muscles surrounding the veins will increase blood flow toward the tourniquet.

Step 5 • Insert the needle or percutaneous catheter with a needle stylet. Affix the extremity to an arm board, and restrain the infant and child, as well as the adult who needs assistance to remain still. Some children who have had frequent IV insertions can control themselves adequately without need for physical restriction and may want to assist during the procedure. In fact, children with hemophilia can be taught to self-insert an IV infusion line when there is a need for them to have a coagulation factor replacement transfusion.

The size of the needle used will depend on the size of the client, the tonicity and turbidity of the substance to be infused, and the proposed length of time for intravenous therapy. With most adults a 20-gauge or 22-gauge needle catheter is used, and with most infants a 25-gauge butterfly scalp vein needle is used. A relatively smaller needle, as compared to vein diameter, decreases the chance of needle-induced phlebitis, since the smaller needle allows more blood to flow around the needle. For use with infants, shorter needles can be maintained more easily. The efficacy of steel needles versus the various plastic catheter counterparts can be assumed only by comparing data from different studies. In studies reviewed by Maki (1976) involving the use of steel needles with 700 subjects, only one patient developed bacteremia, a rate of 0.14%. By comparison, 20 published research projects involving plastic infusion catheters report a systemic infection rate between 0% and 8%. These correlational data demonstrate a need for research studies that actually compare both types of devices, but the data now available tend to support the use of steel needles.

Support the extremity with one hand, pulling the skin down below the proposed needle insertion site to stabilize the vein, and not touching the prepared area. Hold the needle parallel to the vein to be punctured, entering at approximately a 30-degree angle. Once the skin is penetrated, decrease the needle angle and continue pushing the needle toward the vein. As the vein is entered, a change in pressure may be noted, and a "popping" sensation at the needle is felt. Blood return in the needle catheter or syringe will indicate placement within the vein. Release the tourniquet; the needle can then be connected to the prepared IV line, and flow can be established so that a clot does not form at the needle tip. Regulation of the rate can be done once the line is secured.

Step 6 • Secure the IV needle. Taping the needle to the skin should be done with as little tape and dressing material as possible. The needle and line should be secure, yet visible for checking the site for irritation and patency. A small dressing also decreases the discomfort a client may experience because of the dressing itself. Choice of tape should take into consideration the high humidity to which infants and children are exposed in isolettes and mist tents. The following outline gives the steps in securing an IV needle:

1. With a percutaneous catheter, place antibiotic ointment at the insertion site (Fig. 12-1).
2. Cover the insertion site with a plastic bandage. When a butterfly needle is used, anchor the needle first, as described in step 3, below; then apply ointment and bandage over the actual needle point.
3. If a butterfly needle is inserted, affix the needle to the skin, using the wing tips of the butterfly as anchors.
   a. With either the chevron or the H method, first place a piece of ¼-inch tape horizontally over the wings.
   b. With the chevron attachment, place a piece of tape (¼ inch) under the tubing just below the wings, adhesive side up. Take each end of the tape and cross it over the top of the tubing, fastening the tape ends over the wing tips (Fig. 12-2).
   c. Use the H method to place a piece of tape over each wing tip perpendicular to the first piece of tape (Fig. 12-3).

Three components of the line system itself can be extremely significant to the client in maintaining proper flow rate to prevent bacteremia and excessive infusion. The use of any specific type of equipment is not without controversy in patient care. No real consensus is found because few

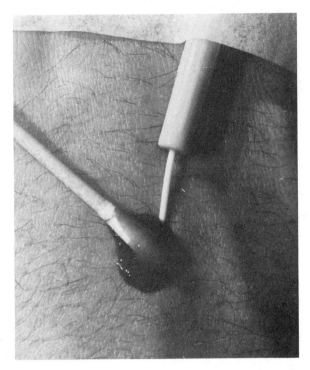

Fig. 12-1. Antibiotic ointment. (Photo by E. David Wood.)

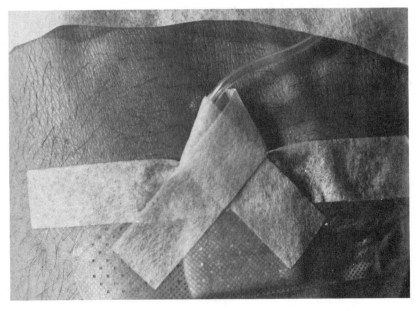

Fig. 12-2. Chevron method. (Photo by E. David Wood.)

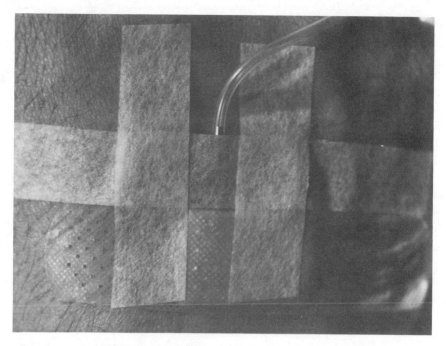

Fig. 12-3. The H method. (Photo by E. David Wood.)

studies have been done to evaluate the pros and cons of any single IV set component. However, strong support for patient safety is found in the use of IV controllers and pumps, in-line final filters, and volume control sets.

IV controllers and pumps

An IV controller is an electronic device that changes the diameter of the IV tubing to maintain a constant infusion rate on gravity-fed infusions. On cursory examination an IV pump looks the same as an IV controller, but its function is different. An IV pump actually applies rhythmic controlled pressure to the IV tubing and provides absolute volume-time control in maintaining an infusion flow. Ziser and associates (1979) determined that IV controllers can maintain a constant rate of infusion. The study compared electronic controllers with the clamps and roller devices packaged with IV tubing and intended to provide set points for maintaining a prescribed IV rate. Factors associated with clamp and roller failure are classified according to such patient-related problems as vein spasm, changes in venous pressure, and movement of the needle or catheter in the line. For example, a crying infant or child can sufficiently raise venous pressure so that IV flow is impeded or obstructed. When crying stops, the preset clamp cannot compensate for the change in venous resistance. Equipment-related factors that affect the clamp or roller functioning are (1) changing pressure in the container, (2) obstructed vents and airway tubes, (3) structural design and material complement of the clamp, which causes unintentional opening, and (4) accommodation to changes in the internal diameter of the tubing after the flow clamp or roller has been adjusted. Ziser and colleagues concluded that since clamps and rollers alone cannot accurately maintain IV flow, controllers should be used.

The IV controllers, although not as precisely accurate as IV pumps, would be preferred in most clinical situations, and they can be vital in preventing rapid accidental overinfusion. The IV pumps can be problematic because, unlike IV controllers, they will continue to pump fluid into an infusion site even if the needle becomes dislodged from the vein.

In-line final filters (Fig. 12-4). Final filters are relatively new IV therapy aids. These filters are considered as primary deterrents to sepsis caused by microorganisms introduced during a client's course of intrave-

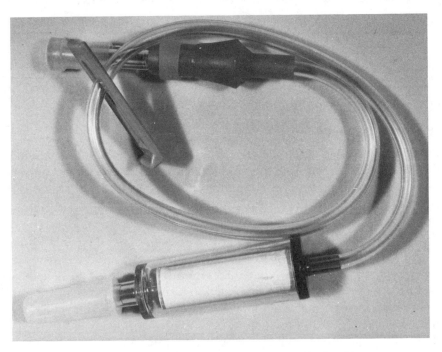

Fig. 12-4. Final filter. (Photo by E. David Wood.)

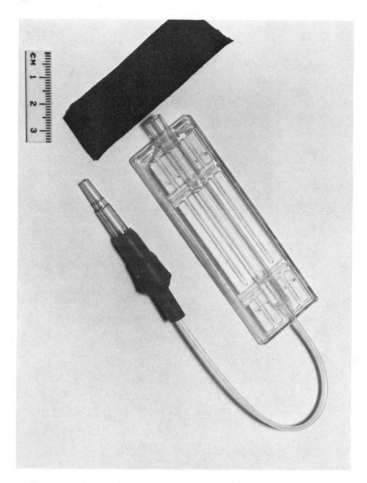

Fig. 12-5. IV filter/air eliminator for use in the parenteral delivery of fluids. (Photo by Gene Luttenberg Photography.)

INTRAVENOUS INFUSION RECORD

Client's name ____D.B.____   IV solution ____D5 .45NS____

Record number ___000000000___   Type of infusion set ___25 ga butterfly___

                                                          approximately

Date ___6-19-81___   24 hour IV fluid requirements ___600 ml___   Hourly rate ___22 ml/hr___

                                               Controller ___X___ Pump _____

Time	Hourly rate	Amount in VCS	Amount infused in last hour	Cumulative amount infused	Amount added to VCS	Fluid deficit or excess	Type of IV solution being used, changes, and initials of nurse
2400	22	0 ml	0 ml	0 ml	30 ml	0	ma
0100	22	8 ml	22 ml	22 ml	8+22 = 30 ml	0	mg
0200	22	8 ml	22 ml	44 ml	8+22 = 30	0	mg
0300	22	8 ml	22 ml	66 ml	8+22 = 30	0	eb
0400	22	8 ml	22 ml	88 ml	8+22 = 30	0	mg
0500	22	8 ml	22 ml	110 ml	8+22 = 30	0	mg
0600	25	20 ml	10 ml	120 ml	20+10 = 30	-12 ml	mg
0700	25	5 ml	25 ml	145 ml	5+25 = 30	-9 ml	mg
0800	25	5 ml	25 ml	170 ml	5+25 = 30	-6 ml	mg
0900	25	5 ml	25 ml	195 ml	5+25 = 30	-3 ml	meb
1000	22	5 ml	25 ml	220 ml	5+25 = 30	0	meb
1100	22	8 ml	22 ml	242 ml	8+22 = 30	0	meb
1200	30	8 ml	22 ml	264 ml	8+27 = 35	0	500 ml D5E75 meb
1300	30	5 ml	30 ml	294 ml	5+30 = 35	0	500 ml D5E75 jb
1400	30	5 ml	30 ml	324 ml	5+40 = 45	0	500 ml D5E75 jb
1500	30	15 ml	30 ml	354 ml	15+30 = 45	0	500 ml D5E75 jb
1600	30	15 ml	30 ml	384 ml	15+30 = 45	0	500 ml D5E75 jb
1700	30	15 ml	30 ml	414 ml	15+30 = 45	0	500 ml D5E75 jb
1800	30	15 ml	30 ml	444 ml	15+30 = 45	0	500 ml D5E75 jb
1900	30	15 ml	30 ml	474 ml	15+30 = 45	0	500 ml D5E75 jb
2000	30	15 ml	30 ml	504 ml	15+30 = 45	0	500 ml D5E75 jb
2100	30	15 ml	30 ml	534 ml	15+20 = 35	0	500 ml D5E75 jb
2200	30	5 ml	30 ml	564 ml	5+30 = 35	0	500 ml D5E75 jb
2300	30	5 ml	30 ml	574 ml	5+30 = 35	0	500 ml D5E75 jb

Fig. 12-6. Sample IV infusion record.

nous therapy. Some filters also eliminate air bubbles that may be inadvertently introduced into the IV system (Fig. 12-5). Contamination can result from the use of improperly manufactured or packaged IV fluids or devices or from errors made by the nursing, anesthesiology, or pharmacy staffs in initiating the use of equipment or manipulating equipment when adding additional tubing or medications. An effectiveness study (Rusho and Bair, 1979) comparing filter use with a controlled sample in which filters were not used clinically demonstrated that the filter group spent an average of 3.35 fewer days in the hospital than the nonfilter group. The nonfilter control group had a greater phlebitis rate. Filters used in the study with 150 patients undergoing orthopedic procedures were 5.0 μm filters and 0.45 μm filters. Also available are 0.22 μm filters, which are capable of essentially stopping all particulates, air, and bacteria introduced into the system. The 0.22 μm filters are deemed more efficient than the larger filters, but they cannot be used with blood byproducts or with lipid emulsions.

Volume control sets. Volume control sets are available from several manufacturers, and they are ideal for infusing a precise volume of fluid and medications. The sets are particularly good for use in providing children with IV fluids.

In addition, volume control sets can be useful for accurately recording the amount of IV fluid infused on an hourly and cumulative basis. Adding IV fluid to the volume control chamber each hour and recording the amount of fluid infused at the end of the hour permits an immediate appraisal of fluid replacement status. The sample recording sheet (Fig. 12-6) illustrates how the nurse documents the infusion, proceeding on an hourly basis.

IV infusion record

Since military time is used in delineating the IV infusion record, the A.M.-P.M. designations are omitted. This type of hourly recording is often used in intensive or coronary care settings. Its use with any person receiving an IV infusion, especially children, provides the assurance that the patient, infusion site, and infusion set are being evaluated frequently.

As seen in Fig. 12-6, D. B. had an IV infusion initiated at midnight, at a rate of 22 ml/hr. Thirty milliliters of IV fluid was added to the volume control set, to allow the nurse a few minutes' leeway at the next hourly check in returning to monitor the client and manipulate the IV equipment.

The infusion was proceeding accurately until 0500 hours (5 A.M.), when the client was transported to the x-ray unit. At 0600 hours, when the client and IV infusion were checked, only 10 ml had been infused since 5 A.M., reflecting a 12 ml deficit.

So that the client would receive the allocated IV fluid, the nurse planned to increase the IV infusion rate by 3 ml/hr over the next 4 hours to make up the fluid loss. By 1000 hours (10 A.M.), the fluid deficit-excess column reflected a balanced state. If the rate had increased and the client had received a fluid excess, the rate could have been gradually decreased to achieve a correct cumulative infusion volume.

At 1200 hours the IV rate and solution were changed. This change is reflected on the record. Changes throughout the day can be visualized at a glance. The information on the record can provide the health care team with an up-to-date account of the type and amount of fluids the client is receiving and can do so in a manner that is expedient and enhances both accountability and client safety.

Generally speaking, safety needs dictate that infants under 1 year of age should have a 250 ml bottle or less of IV fluid attached to their IV lines and that children under the age of 16 years should have a 500 ml bottle of fluid connected to their IV lines. Adults can be infused by means of a 1000 ml bottle of IV fluid, depending on the rate of IV flow required. The risk of overhydration in babies and young children because of accidental overinfusion is of great concern. The safety needs of the client mandate using an IV bag or bottle with the smallest practical amount of volume, considering hourly IV flow rate. Over time this practice may eliminate waste, since IV fluids may be changed frequently during the acute phase of an illness to reflect the changing physiologic state of the client. Using the smallest bottle in conjunction with a volume control set and IV controller conceivably triples the protection against accidental overhydration afforded the infant, child, or adult.

Recommendations regarding the need to change all or part of an IV setup are summarized in Table 12-5. Many of these recommendations are made by the U.S. Center for Disease Control, in Atlanta, or the National Coordinating Committee on Large Volume Parenterals. Individual hospitals may use these recommendations as guidelines in planning and implementing infusion policies for their individual settings. Certainly, IV therapy is an adjunct to patient care that is nearly indispensable in maintaining or stabilizing a patient. Although its expense is justifiable, nurses need to be cognizant of the fact that an average IV setup, from bottle to butterfly needle, costs nearly $30.00 (December, 1979 prices). Thus changes made in the entire setup or its parts because of any type of negligence are expensive to the client not only in terms of personal trauma and increased risk of sepsis but also in monetary terms.

Table 12-5. Guidelines for changing components of IV administration set*

Change(s), if any, in IV setup	Status of patient or infusion	Time
Change dressing and taping	Normal	Every 24 hours
Change administration set, filter, venipuncture device, and venipuncture site	Normal	Every 48 hours
Change container	Normal, with fluid in container nearly depleted	Any time
Change administration set, container, dressing, filter, taping, venipuncture device, and venipunture site	*Any of the following:* Allergic reaction to ointment Blood clot in venipuncture device Deep hematoma Defect in venipuncture device Disconnection in tubing (tubing contaminated) Infiltration Localized infection Phlebitis	Any time
Change administration set, container, dressing, filter, and taping	Crack or puncture in container	Any time
Change administration set, dressing, filter, and taping	*Either of the following:* Defect in control clamp Saturated filter	Any time
Change dressing and taping (as indicated)	*Any of the following:* Allergic reaction to tape Crimp in IV loop Obstructive tape	Any time
Add IV pump or controller	*Either of the following:* Circulatory overload (no delivery of fluid in excess of plan) Delivery of fluid in excess of plan (no circulatory overload)	Any time
No material change in setup	Disconnection in tubing (tubing not contaminated) Superficial hematoma (bruise)	Any time

*From Cohen, S.: Am. J. Nurs. **79:**1278, July 1979. Copyright, 1979, American Journal of Nursing Company. Reproduced with permission from the American Journal of Nursing.

HYPERALIMENTATION

The need to maintain a positive nitrogen balance during illness has led to the development of a subspecialty area in IV fluid administration. Several distinct methods of nutritional IV intervention are available, including (1) peripheral vein infusion of protein-sparing formulations, (2) peripheral or central vein infusion of total parenteral nutrition (TPN) solutions, and (3) central vein infusion for IV hyperalimentation (IVH). The following chart summarizes the relative compositions of each type of solution.

Protein-sparing solutions	*Intravenous hyperalimentation*	*Total parenteral nutrition*
Amino acids 400 to 600 kcal/24 hr	Amino acids Dextrose (25%) 2,400 to 3,000 kcal/24 hr	Amino acids Fats Dextrose (5% to 10%) 2,400 to 3,000 kcal/24 hr

The amino acid component of the hyperalimentation solution supplies 170 kcal/liter, and the amount of 5% solution infused should not exceed 2 liters in 6 hours. Nursing actions regarding its use include observations for anaphylactic shock, convulsions, nausea, vomiting, abdominal pain, elevated temperature, and edema at the infusion site. Protein hydrolysate should not be used if the patient is in an acidotic state, and benefits must outweigh the risks for those with severe renal or liver disease.

A fat emulsion such as Intralipid can supply up to 60% of the calories in TPN solutions. Intralipid, 10%, is most frequently used, but 20% fat emulsions will be used more often as development and marketing progress. Fat emulsions are composed of soybean oil emulsions and purified egg phospholipids in glycerol in water. Because of the relatively large size of the fat particles, an in-line filter cannot be used with this preparation. The fine fat particles can aggregate if the solution is agitated or shaken. Aside from the amino acid–dextrose solution with which fat emulsions are mixed, nothing else should be added to lipid emulsions, including other IV solutions, medications, blood, or electrolytes.

Baseline data regarding the patient's status enable the nurse to monitor vital signs during Intralipid administration and correctly evaluate changes in pulse, respiration, blood pressure, and temperature. Reactions to fat emulsions may include chills, fever, diaphoresis, rubor, dyspnea, cyanosis, allergic responses, thoracic or flank pain, nausea, vomiting, headache, bradycardia, tachycardia, increased ocular pressure, vertigo, drowsiness, or thrombophlebitis. These reactions may be present in the initial phase of fat emulsion therapy, but cumulative reactions may also develop. The nurse must be alert to signs of the fat overload syndrome, which is characterized by headache, irritability, low-grade fever, abdominal pain, nausea, anemia, and coagulopathy. Abdominal palpation may reveal an enlarged liver and spleen. Baseline laboratory data for a patient who will receive Intralipid should include liver function studies, determinations of serum cholesterol and serum triglyceride levels, and the results of testing for serum lipemia. These tests should be repeated weekly to assess response to treatment. In infants and children, checking for serum lipemia is recommended on a daily basis. Serum lipemia is measured by checking the fat in a capillary tube after the blood cells and serum have been separated.

Dextrose solutions used in combination with amino acid and lipid preparations vary in concentration from 5% to 25%. The additive advantage of amino acids and lipids increases the total caloric input and decreases total fluid volume. Dextrose solutions alone significantly increase total fluid and would predispose most clients to fluid overload because of the fluid-to-calorie ratio of dextrose solutions. Dextrose solutions infused faster than 500 μg/kg/hr would surpass the renal tubular maximum (T_m) for glucose and cause glycosuria. Testing the urine in patients receiving hyperalimentation for sugar and acetone is done to evaluate renal function. Solutions with dextrose concentrations greater than 10% are especially irritating to the veins and may predispose the patient to phlebitis. Peripheral venous irritation can be prevented by infusing the dextrose solution into the vena cava. In addition to collecting data regarding glycosuria, the nurse should also monitor the patient for transient reactive hyperinsulinism, which is characterized by weakness, apprehension, diaphoresis, hypotension, disorientation, and convulsions.

CONCLUSION

The various IV therapy modalities change as quickly as new technology of administration and new solutions are introduced into practice. Patient outcomes are greatly affected by the knowledge and skill of the nurse in providing administration of IV preparations that is skillful and safe and will therefore prevent infection, phlebitis, thrombophlebitis, overhydration, and known complications of IV incompatibilities.

References

Acute diarrhoea in childhood, Ciba Foundation Symposium, 42, Amsterdam, 1976, Elsevier Scientific Publishing Co.

Alvarez, R., editor: The kidney in pregnancy, New York, 1976, John Wiley & Sons.

Anderson, B.: Regulation of body fluids, Annu. Rev. Physiol. **39:**185-200, 1977.

Assali, S., editor: Pathophysiology of gestation, vol. 1, New York, 1972, Academic Press.

Bauman, J. W., Jr., and Chinard, F. P.: Renal function, St. Louis, 1975, The C. V. Mosby Co.

Bland, J.: Clinical metabolism of body water and electrolytes, Philadelphia, 1963, W. B. Saunders Co.

Bickel, H., and Sterr, J., editors: Inborn errors of calcium and bone metabolism, Baltimore, 1976, University Park Press.

Brackemyre, P., and Schreiner, R.: Late metabolic acidosis of the premature infant, J. Am. Diet. Assoc. **72:**298-301, 1978.

Colley, R., Wilson, J., and Mabel, D.: Meeting patients' nutritional needs with hyperalimentation, Nursing '79, **9:**50-52, 1979.

Davenport, H. W.: The ABC of acid-base chemistry: the elements of physiological blood-gas chemistry for medical students and physicians, ed. 6, Chicago, 1974, University of Chicago Press.

Dennis, V., Stead, W., and Myers, J.: Renal handling of phosphate and calcium, Annu. Rev. Physiol. **41:**257-272, 1979.

Dethier, V. G.: The taste of salt, Am. Sci. **65:**744-751, 1977.

Final in-line filters, Am. J. Nurs. **79:**1272-1273, 1979.

Finch, C., and Hayflick, L.: Handbook of the biology of aging, New York, 1977, Van Nostrand Reinhold Co.

Fitzsimmons, J.: Angiotensin, thirst, and sodium appetite: retrospect and prospect, Fed. Proc. **37:**2669-2675, 1978.

Ford, J. D., and Haworth, J. C.: The fecal excretion of sugars in children, J. Pediatr. **63:**988-990, Nov., 1963.

Givens, J., editor: Endocrine causes of menstrual disorders, Chicago, 1977, Year Book Medical Publishers.

Grant, M. M., and Kubo, W. M.: Assessing a patient's hydration status, Am. J. Nurs. **75:**1307-1311, Aug., 1975.

Groër, M. E., and Omachi, A.: Inhibition of sodium extrusion from intact human erythrocytes by phosopholipase A and lysophospholipids, Fed. Proc. **33:**366, 1974.

Groër, M. E., and Shekleton, M. E.: Basic pathophysiology: a conceptual approach, St. Louis, 1979, The C. V. Mosby Co.

278

Hamilton, H., editor: Monitoring fluid and electrolytes precisely, Horsham, Pa., 1978, Nursing '79 Books, Intermed Communications.

Howells, E. M.: Managing fluids and electrolytes in surgical patients, Geriatrics **32:**100-101, 1977.

Jacobson, N. T.: How to administer those tricky lipid emulsions, RN **42:**63-64, 1979.

James, D. K., Dryburgh, E. H., and Chiswich, M. L.: Foot length: a new and potentially useful measurement in the neonate, Arch. Dis. Child. **54:**226-230, 1979.

Katz, F., and Romgh, P.: Plasma aldosterone and renin activity during the menstrual cycle, J. Clin. Endocrinol. Metab. **34:**819-821, 1972.

Kee, J. L., and Gregory, A. P.: The ABC's and mEq's of fluid imbalance in children, Nursing '74 **4:**28-36, June, 1974.

Lawson, M., Bottino, J. C., and McCredie, K. B.: Long-term IV therapy: a new approach, Am. J. Nurs. **79:**1100-1103, 1979.

Lim, J. C.: Technique for microbiological testing of intravenous solutions and administration sets, Am. J. Hosp. Pharm. **36:**1202-1204, 1979.

Lindeman, R. D.: Application of fluid and electrolyte balance principles to the older patient. In Reichel, W., editor: Clinical aspects of aging, Baltimore, 1978, The Williams & Wilkins Co.

Maki, D. G.: Preventing infection in intravenous therapy, Hosp. Pract. **11:**95-104, April, 1976.

Maki, D. G., Weise, M. S., and Sarafin, H. W.: A semiquantitative culture method for identifying intravenous catheter-related infection, N. Engl. J. Med. **296:**1305-1309, June, 1977.

Maxwell, M., and Kleeman, C.: Clinical disorders of fluid and electrolyte metabolism, New York, 1972, McGraw-Hill Book Co.

McGrath, B.: Fluids, electrolytes, and replacement therapy in pediatric nursing, MCN **5:**58-62, 1980.

McKinley, M., Blaine, E., and Denton, D.: Brain osmoreceptors, cerebrospinal fluid electrolyte composition, and thirst, Brain Res. **70:**532-537, 1974.

Mead Johnson Symposium on Perinatal and Developmental Medicine, No. 10: Developmental aspects of fluid and electrolyte homeostasis, Marco Island, Fla., 1976, Mead Johnson Laboratories.

Metheny, N. A., and Snively, W. D.: Perioperative fluids and electrolytes, Am. J. Nurs. **78:**840-845, 1978.

Millam, D. A.: How to insert an IV, Am. J. Nurs. **79:**1268-1271, 1979.

Mountcastle, V. B., editor: Medical physiology, ed. 14, St. Louis, 1980, The C. V. Mosby Co.

Nichols, B. L., and others: Anomalies of the regulation of salt and water in protein-calorie malnutrition. In Gardner, L. I., and Amacher, P., editors: Endocrine aspects of malnutrition, Santa Inez, Calif., 1973, The Kroc Foundation.

Phipps, D.: Metals and metabolism, Oxford, 1976, Clarendon Press.

Pritchard, J., and MacDonald, P.: Williams' obstetrics, ed. 15, New York, 1976, Appleton-Century-Crofts.

Programmed instruction: Fundamentals of IV maintenance, Am. J. Nurs. **79:**1274-1287, 1979.

Reid, I.: The brain renin-angiotensin system: a critical analysis, Fed. Proc. **38:**2255-2259, 1979.

Rose, D. B.: Clinical physiology of acid-base and electrolyte disorders, New York, 1977, McGraw-Hill Book Co.

Rusho, W. J., and Bair, J. N.: Effect of filtration on complications of postoperative intravenous therapy, Am. J. Hosp. Pharm. **36:**1355-1356, 1979.

Schwartz, V. D., and Abraham, G.: Corticosterone and aldosterone levels during the menstrual cycle, Obstet. Gynecol. **45:**339-342, 1975.

Smith, C., and Nelson, N.: The physiology of the newborn infant, ed. 4, Springfield, Ill., 1976, Charles C Thomas, Publisher.

Stern, R.: Pathophysiologic basis for symptomatic treatment of fever, Pediatrics **59:**92-98, 1977.

Stricker, E. M.: The renin-angiotensin system and thirst—some unanswered questions, Fed. Proc. **37:**2704-2710, 1978.

Thurau, K., editor: Kidney and urinary tract physiology, vol. 2, Baltimore, 1976, University Park Press.

Tilkian, S. M., Conover, M. B., and Tilkian, A. G.: Clinical implications of laboratory tests, ed. 2, St. Louis, 1979, The C. V. Mosby Co.

Trunkey, D. D.: Review of current concepts in fluid and electrolyte management, Heart Lung **4:**115-121, 1975.

Twombley, M.: The shift into third space, Nursing '78 **8:**38-41, June, 1978.

Weil, W. B., and Bailie, M. D.: Fluid and electrolyte metabolism in infants and children: a unified approach, New York, 1977, Grune & Stratton.

White, S. J.: IV fluids and electrolytes: how to head off the risks, RN **42:**60-63, 1979.

Winters, R., editor: The body fluids in pediatrics, Boston, 1973, Little, Brown & Co.

Ziser, M., Feezor, M., and Skolaut, M. W.: Regulating intravenous fluid flow: controller versus clamps, Am. J. Hosp. Pharm. **36:**1090-1094, 1979.

Table of normal values

Blood chemistries

Albumin   4.3-5.6 gm/dl
Ammonia   102 μg/dl
Calcium   9.0-11.5 mg/dl
CO_2 combining power   25-33 mmole/liter
Chloride   95-106 mEq/liter
Cholesterol   220 ± 50 mg/dl
Copper   90-150 μg/dl
Creatine   0.6-1.5 mg/dl
Creatinine clearance   97-123 ml/min
Fluoride   less than 0.05 mg/dl
Glucose   70-110 mg/dl
Iodine   4.0-8.0 μg/dl (protein bound)
Iron   50-150 μg/dl
Lactic acid   0.6-1.8 mEq/liter
Osmolarity   280-295 mOsm/liter
Pco_2 Arterial blood = 40 mm Hg
Po_2 Arterial blood = 95-100 mm Hg
pH   7.35-7.45
Potassium   3.8-4.1 mEq/liter
Protein (total)   6.0-8.4 gm/dl
Renin activity   1.1 ± 0.8 ng/ml/hr
Sodium   136-142 mEq/liter
Sulfate   0.5-1.5 mEq/liter
Urea nitrogen (BUN)   5-25 mg/dl
Zinc   50-150 μg/dl

Urine chemistries and renal function

Calcium   100-250 mg/24 hr
Chloride   110-250 mEq/24 hr
Creatine   less than 100 mg/24 hr

Glomerular filtration rate   120 ml/min
Lead   less than 100 μg/24 hr
Magnesium   6.0-8.5 mEq/24 hr
pH   4.6-7.8
Phosphorus   0.9-1.3 gm/24 hr
Potassium   40-80 mEq/24 hr
Renal blood flow   1200 ml/min
Sodium   80-180 mEq/24 hr
Specific gravity   1.001-1.035 (average 1.010)
Titratable acidity   20-50 mEq/24 hr
Urea   6-17 gm/24 hr
Volume   600-1600 ml/24 hr

Hematology

Hematocrit: male 40%-45%; female 38%-47%
Hemoglobin: male 13.5-18.0 gm/dl; female 12-16 gm/dl

Index